SHEEP AND GOAT DISEASES

Veterinary Book for Farmers and Smallholders

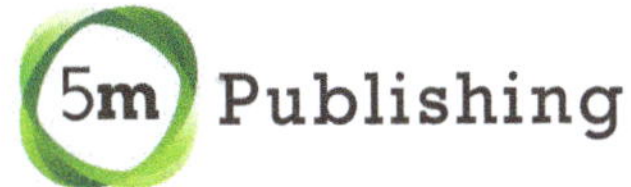

SHEEP AND GOAT DISEASES

Veterinary Book for Farmers and Smallholders

4th Edition

Johannes Winkelmann

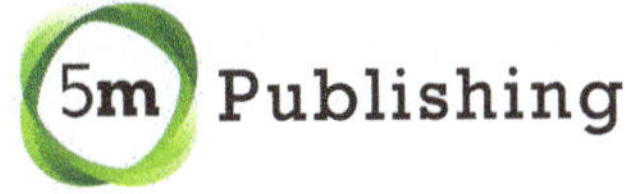

Fourth German language edition published 2014
This edition published by 5m Publishing 2016

Authorized translation of the fourth German language edition of Winkelmann Johannes, Schaf- und Ziegenkrankheiten © 2014 by Eugen Ulmer KG, Stuttgart, Germany

Published by
5M Publishing Ltd,
Benchmark House,
8 Smithy Wood Drive,
Sheffield, S35 1QN, UK
Tel: +44 (0) 1234 81 81 80
www.5mpublishing.com

A Catalogue record for this book is available from the British Library

ISBN 9781789184136

Book layout by
Keystroke, Neville Lodge, Tettenhall, Wolverhampton

Photos by Johannes Winkelmann; Dr. C. Koch, Münster; K. A. Linklater, Edinburgh; F. Neiß, Cologne; Dr. G. Steng, Stuttgart; H. Weischet, Velbert; Dr. W. Adams, Münster; W. Baumeister, Stuttgart; Prof. Dr. H. Bostedt, Gießen; Thume, O., Kaisersbach

Illustrations by Brigitte Zwickel-Noelle

Important note: The names of drugs which are also registered trademarks are not specifically identified as such in this book. Referring to a product by its registered trademark does not imply that the name is a free product name. Brand names are mentioned only by way of example. The greatest possible care has been taken with regard to the drug dosages etc. indicated in this book. However, readers are advised to check the manufacturer's package insert.

Contents

Foreword to the 4th edition

This book for sheep and goat keepers, first published almost exactly 19 years ago, is now in its fourth edition. It has been revised to take account of developments in sheep and goat husbandry and to reflect advances and limitations in terms of medication which are relevant to both keepers and vets. It also considers and explains the significance of new information on certain diseases (such as Johne's disease and Q fever) that has come to light in recent years as a result of scientific investigation. Sections on bluetongue and Schmallenberg virus infection have been added.

Something that has not changed is the fact that sheep and goats are kept by different types of people from different walks of life. On the one hand there are full-time sheep and goat farmers, while other people keep their animals as a sideline or hobby. What both groups share is a concern for the animals in their charge and their efforts to obtain as much information as they can about the keeping, husbandry, care and health of their animals.

Like its predecessors, this new edition is designed to enable full-time farmers, part-time keepers and hobbyists alike to look after their animals' health, to identify diseases promptly and to take appropriate measures to prevent losses. The focus is on identifying diseases and on the measures we can take to prevent them.

In its present form, of course, the book cannot and does not aim to list every single disease that may affect sheep and goats.

It incorporates the latest information on the treatment of worm diseases and lists the wormers that are currently available. It also explains the problems associated with dispensing veterinary medicines to sheep and goat keepers. It outlines the difficulties involved in controlling worm diseases in organic sheep and goat farming. I would like to thank the sheep and goat farmers, and veterinary colleagues, who supplied illustrations for the book (H. Weischet, Velbert; R. Vinbrüx, now Oamaru, New Zealand; F. Neiß, Cologne; G. Steng, Stuttgart; W. Adams, C. Koch, P. Heimberg, Münster; M. Ganter, Hanover; K. Voigt, Munich), and those who gave up their time and effort to help me to obtain appropriate images (R. Herschmann, Cologne and E. Schwarz, St Augustin).

Special thanks are due to my wife for her generous support, patience and understanding during the preparation of the manuscript.

J. Winkelmann

1

Healthy sheep and goats

Sheep were first domesticated around 8,000 years BC, making them one of our earliest farm animals. They are now the world's second most common species of farm animal, and their importance as providers of wool and meat remains undisputed.

In the UK, home-produced lamb has recently been gaining in popularity, and sheep and goats are increasingly being used in landscape conservation to farm and maintain extensive pasture land.

Besides full-time farmers, more and more people are keeping sheep and goats as a hobby, owning just a few animals and making products (milk, cheese) for their own use or for sale. As a result, keeping sheep and goats healthy is becoming increasingly important – partly in order to avoid transmitting disease to humans.

Anatomy and normal physiological functions

The next few pages contain some basic information about the anatomy and physiological functions of healthy sheep and goats.

The musculoskeletal system consists of the skeleton and muscles. The **skeleton** can be divided into the head, neck, body and limbs. The skeleton also includes the teeth, which can be used to determine the approximate age of the animal. The **chest cavity** is defined by the thoracic vertebrae above, the ribs on either side and the breastbone below, and contains the **heart** and **lungs**. These two crucial organs are perfectly protected by their surrounding bony cage. The chest cavity is separated from the abdominal cavity by the **diaphragm**, which is the most important respiratory muscle.

The **abdominal cavity** contains the internal organs or 'viscera': the **liver**, which is the body's primary metabolic organ, the **kidneys**, which produce urine and play an important role in detoxification, and the **spleen**, which is part of the immune system. This cavity also holds the digestive organs: the **rumen**, **reticulum**, **omasum**, **abomasum**, **small intestine** and **large intestine**. These organs are surrounded by the lumbar vertebrae above and by the abdominal muscles on the other three sides. These muscles enable the abdominal cavity to expand to an extent, helping it to adjust to different degrees of fullness of the gastrointestinal tract – or of the uterus in pregnant females.

After the abdominal cavity comes the pelvic cavity, which contains the **bladder**, the **male** or **female reproductive organs** and the **rectum**.

Normal physiological data in sheep and goats

	Sheep	Goat
Body temperature	38.5–39.5 °C	39–40 °C
Pulse	60–80 beats/minute	77–89 beats/minute
Respiratory rate (resting)	10–20 breaths/minute	15–25 breaths/minute
Sexual maturity	5–8 months	5–8 months
Oestrus period (seasonal breeds)	September–February	September–February
Duration of oestrus	30–36 hours	12–48 hours
Oestrus cycle	18–21 days	19–21 days
Pregnancy	150 (145–154) days	150 (146–154) days

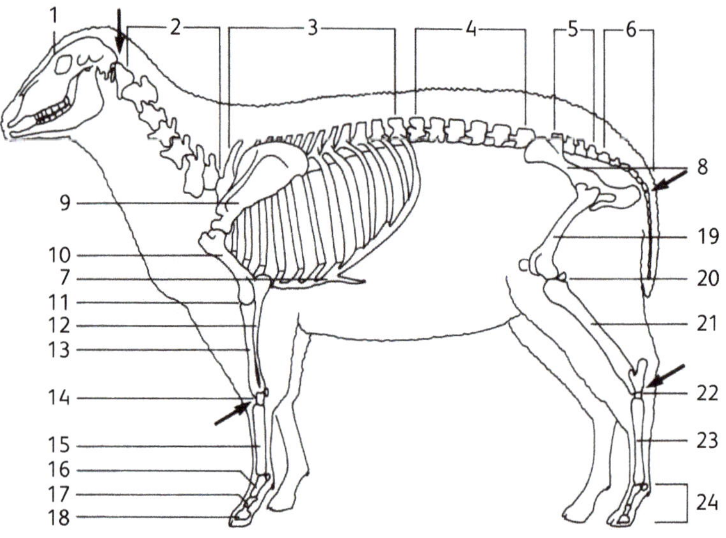

1 Skull
2 7 cervical vertebrae
3 13 thoracic vertebrae with one rib each
4 lumbar vertebrae
5 4 sacral vertebrae
6 3 – 24 caudal vertebrae
7 Breastbone
8 Pelvis
9 Shoulder blade
10 Humerus
11 Elbow joint
12 Ulna
13 Radius
14 Carpal (knee) joint
15 Metacarpal bone
16 First phalanx
17 Second phalanx
18 Third phalanx
19 Femur
20 Stifle joint
21 Tibia
22 Tarsal joint
23 Metacarpal bone
24 Phalanges as for fore foot

➔ Carcass cutting points

The skeleton of the sheep.

Dentition formula in small ruminants

	Incisors	Canines	Premolars	Molars
Upper jaw	Dental plate		3	3
Lower jaw	3	1	3	3
Milk teeth	0–21 days	3–4 weeks	0–4 weeks	Not present
2nd dentition	1–3 years	3–4 years	1–2 years	Eruption by age 2

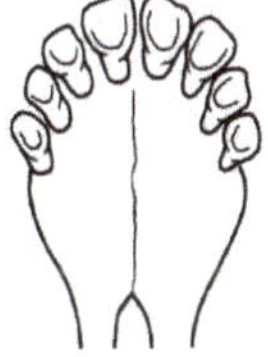

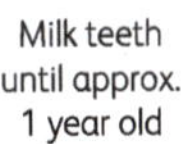
Milk teeth until approx. 1 year old

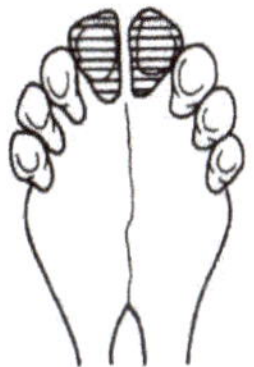
Central incisor change at age 1 – 1.5

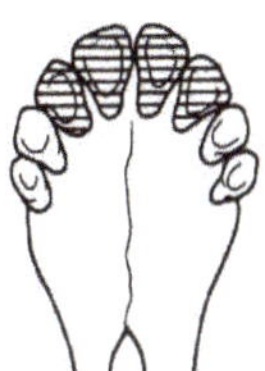
Middle incisor change at age 2 – 2.5

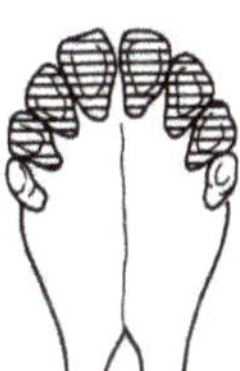
Lateral incisor change at age 2.5 – 3

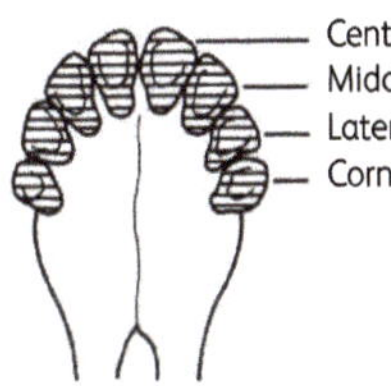

Corner incisor change at age 3.5 – 4

Age-dependent incisor change in the sheep.
The remaining teeth are shaded.

Different feed rations for empty ewes and ewes in early pregnancy (von Korn, 2001)

Feed	Different feed rations (kg/animal/day)							
	1	2	3	4	5	6	7	8
Pasture grass (late pasture)	6.0	–	–	–	–	–	–	–
Hay (good quality)	–	1.0	0.7	–	–	–	–	–
Hay (moderate quality)	–	–	–	1.0	1.0	1.5	1.8	–
Grass silage (30 % DM)	–	–	–	–	2.0	–	–	–
Maize silage (21 % DM)	–	–	3.0	–	–	–	–	4.0
Beet leaf silage (20 % DM)	–	–	–	2.5	–	–	–	–
Fodder beet	–	2.2	–	–	–	0.4	–	–
Straw	–	–	–	–	–	–	–	0.7
Mineral feed (with vitamins)	–	0.02	0.02	0.02	0.02	0.02	0.02	0.02
Ration contents:								
– DM (kg)	1.6	1.2	1.3	1.4	1.2	1.6	1.5	1.5
– Crude fibre	35	21	19	26	32	40	36	32
– Digestible protein (g)	90	94	85	79	92	66	76	82
– Starch units (SU)	660	610	670	643	580	490	488	628

DM = dry matter.

Recommended daily nutritional and mineral requirements in ewes (von Korn, 2001)

	Weight (kg)	Dry matter (kg)	Digestible crude protein (g)	Starch units (SU)	Ratio CP: SU (1: ...)	Ca (g)	P (g)	Na (g)
Maintenance	60	1.2	66	480	7.2	7.5	5.5	1.5
	75	1.5	80	570	7.2	7.5	5.5	1.5
Mating	60	1.5	110	760	6.9	10.0	7.0	2.0
	75	1.8	120	850	6.9	10.0	7.0	2.0
Early pregnancy	60	1.5	80	550	6.7	8.5	6.0	2.0
	75	1.8	95	640	6.7	8.5	6.0	2.0
Late pregnancy[1]	60	1.5	145	800	5.5	15.0	7.5	2.0
	75	1.8	160	890	5.5	15.0	7.5	2.0
Lactation[2]								
Single lamb	60	2.0	260	1140	4.3	17.0	9.0	2.0
	75	2.2	280	1230	4.3	17.0	9.0	2.0
Twins[3]	60	2.0	370	1570	4.3	20.0	10.0	2.5
	75	2.2	390	1650	4.3	20.0	10.0	2.5

1 Ewe carrying a single lamb.
2 During the first half of lactation (8 weeks).
3 With supplementary feeding of lambs.

Nutritional requirements of goats: maintenance and performance levels (recommended figures, from Späth and Thume, 2005)

	Dry matter (kg)	NEL (MJ)	Crude protein (g)	Calcium (g)	Phosphorus (g)
Maintenance req.s (60 kg)	1.0–1.2	6.3	70	4.5	2.8
Building of body reserves	1.8	8.5	125	6.0	4.0
4th month of pregnancy	1.9	9.0	140	7.5	4.5
5th month of pregnancy	2.1	12.3	220	8.8	6.0
To produce: 1 kg milk	2.0	9.2	145	6.5	4.2
2 kg milk	2.2	12.1	220	8.5	5.6
3 kg milk	2.5	15.0	295	10.5	7.0
4 kg milk	2.8	17.9	370	12.5	8.4
5 kg milk	3.0	20.8	445	14.5	9.8
6 kg milk	3.2	23.7	520	16.5	11.2

The dentition formula is the number of teeth in one side (or quadrant) of the mouth. To calculate the total number of teeth, multiply the dentition formula by two, for both upper and lower jaw, and add the resulting figures together. Sheep and goats have a total of 32 teeth (including 20 milk teeth).

The animal can be aged on the basis of the number of permanent incisors.

Nutrition

Animals should be fed according to their **maintenance requirements** and **performance requirements**. Maintenance requirements serve to maintain physiological functions, while performance requirements meet additional demands placed on the animal during growth, pregnancy and milk production.

The most important requirement for sheep and goats is an ample supply of good-quality hay and straw, which should ideally be provided *ad libitum*. The high crude fibre content of this fodder helps to prevent digestive disorders and is ideally suited to ruminants.

Besides food, a good supply of **water** is essential. An indoor-housed sheep fed on coarse and fresh fodder needs 1.5 to 3 litres of water per day; a sheep fed on hay and concentrates needs 5 to 7 litres. Lactating ewes need even more because they require larger volumes of liquid in order to produce milk.

Drinkers and feed troughs should be cleaned regularly.

Feeding of dams

The feed rations given in this book for empty ewes and ewes in early pregnancy, late pregnancy and lactation are based on the recommendations in von Korn (2001). In the same way as for sheep, feeding requirements for goats should be tailored to their current performance status. Goats need to build body reserves during the 'dry period' in order to be in good nutritional condition when they kid. But they should not be overfed either. Late pregnancy is the right time to start laying the foundations for the higher-energy lactation diet. Gradually increasing the concentrate ration allows the rumen to adapt to this type of feed, so that concentrates can continue to be given after lambing without triggering any metabolic disorders.

Feeding of lambs

How lambs are fed depends on how they are reared.

In **natural rearing**, lambs stay with their mothers for 12 to 16 weeks, consuming only mother's milk for the first week. From the third week, they are given hay *ad lib.* and gradually increasing amounts of concentrates with a protein/starch ratio of 1:5 (von Korn, 2001). This gradual increase is important in order to avoid the risk of 'pulpy kidney' disease.

The suckling lamb's rumen becomes functional from week seven.

Concentrate rations:
Week 3: 50 g,
Week 5: 150 g,
Week 7: 300 g,
Week 9: 400 g.

Early weaning means introducing lambs to concentrates, hay and water earlier than normal. From week 2, in addition to mother's milk, they are gradually introduced to the new feeding conditions. The early intake of crude fibre stimulates rumen development. Early-weaned lambs receive more concentrates

Nutritional requirements and development of kids intended for breeding (Späth and Thume, 2005)

Age	Daily requirements crude protein (g)	NEL (MJ)	Daily weight gain (g)	Live weight (kg)	
Birth	–	–	–	3.5	
1st month	130	4.2	200	9.5	
2nd month	135	4.9	180	14.9	
3rd month	135	5.6	160	19.7	
4th month	130	6.0	140	23.9	
5th month	125	6.2	120	27.5	
6th month	120	6.4	110	30.8	
7th month	120	6.8	110	34.1	Mating
8th month	125	7.0	100	37.1	Mating
9th month	130	7.4	100	40.1	
10th month	140	8.1	90	42.8	
11th month	150	9.0	90	45.5	
12th month	163	10.0	80	47.9	
13th month	180	10.9	70	50.0	
14th month	195	11.8	60	51.8	Lambing

(around 200 g more per animal per day) than lambs reared with their mothers. Lambs should weigh at least 14 kg on weaning.

Around a week before weaning, the dams' feed ration should be cut back in order to reduce their milk yield. In **motherless rearing**, lambs are given colostrum for the first two days (this is vital as colostrum contains special antibodies which protect against disease). They are then weaned and fed milk replacer from a lamb feeder; concentrates and hay are also provided.

Motherless rearing entails a high risk of disease, as the lambs often do not receive enough colostrum and diseases are easily transmitted via the rubber teats of the feeder. Hygiene, disinfection and close observation of lambs increase the keeper's workload but are essential in order to spot diseases promptly.

The different types of **fattening** – including creep feeding and pasture, feed lot and concentrate finishing – are not discussed here. Readers are advised to consult the relevant literature (e.g. von Korn, 2001).

Until they are four weeks old, all **kids** receive the same food, i.e. mother's milk. Then they are divided into breeding and fattening groups. Kids to be used for breeding now need to start eating roughage. Concentrates and hay are provided to meet their nutritional needs. A good supply of water is essential:

- a 10-week old kid needs around three litres of fluid per day.

Goat fattening is profitable up to a live weight of 25 kg. This means that it is essentially based on milk fattening, with the kids receiving milk replacer. This does not apply in the

UK though. Many male kids are destroyed at birth because it is not economic to rear them.

Sheep keeping

In sheep and goat keeping, a general distinction is made between hill flocks and paddock keeping.

Hill flocks

In this method of husbandry, the shepherd – assisted by herding dogs – needs to be able to drive the flock along roads and paths in a controlled way without endangering traffic. The sheep have the opportunity to eat fresh fodder twice a day. In between, they need to have time to ruminate and digest. The shepherd must take care to get the sheep gradually used to the different types of fodder, in order to avoid digestive disorders and bloat.

Depending on which pastures are available, the sheep will be tended closely or allowed to roam and penned in the intervening rest periods. Each animal should have around 1.4 m^2 of space in the pen. Sheep are generally robust creatures, which makes them well suited to living outdoors all year round.

In the case of hill flocks, the availability of grazing pastures determines where they go. Early summer pastures (from April to July) are low-yielding grassland. On summer pastures, sheep help to conserve the landscape by grazing protected areas.

Paddock keeping

In this method of husbandry, sheep are kept on pastures with permanent or moveable fencing. The importance of paddock keeping is growing year on year because:

- it suits part-time farmers,
- parcels of land can be used as they become free,
- animals do not need to be tended as closely as those in hill flocks.

Continuous monitoring of worm burdens and targeted worming programmes are vital in sheep and goats kept in paddocks.

Goat keeping

Keepers of goats should consider the unique traits peculiar to this species.

Goats are sociable animals. They need the companionship of fellow goats, other animals or people. Changes in their surroundings are immediately noticed and can trigger changes in behaviour. Goats sold to a new owner sometimes display homesickness, in the form of continual bleating and a drop in feed and water intake. Older goats and bucks are particularly sensitive. If sheep and goats are kept together, the goats will automatically take control. Goats, especially bucks, will ram and head-butt each other during fights over pecking order. Horned and hornless (polled) goats should never be kept together because the horned animals will exploit their dominant position. Compared with hornless breeds, horned goats cause much more damage and wear to buildings, equipment and fences.

Goats prefer to rest in high places from where they can keep a closer eye on their surroundings and respond quickly to strange noises and movements.

Indoor keeping

Most dairy goats are kept indoors all year round. The single most important reason for housing commercial dairy herds of up

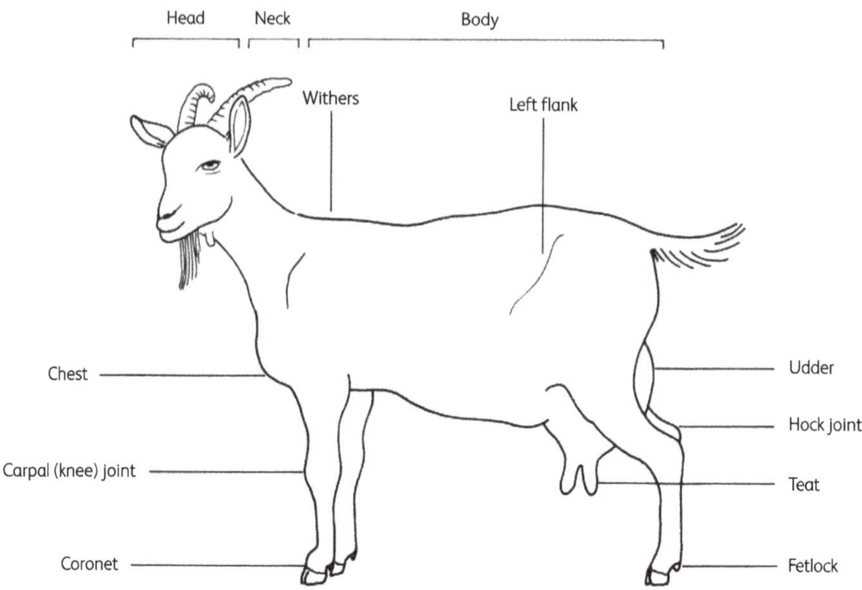

Anatomy of the goat

to 5,000 is to control gut worm infestations, to which goats remain susceptible throughout their lives. In organic farming, however, an outdoor run is a legal requirement. **Tethering** offers the advantages of controlled feeding for the individual goat and smaller space requirements per animal. A chain and leather collar are used to tie the animals up within easy reach of feed troughs and drinkers. A significant drawback of this method is the lack of freedom of movement. As a consequence, it is no longer recommended in goats that are active, lively animals and it is currently illegal in the UK to do so.

A **loose house** gives goats the freedom of movement they need. Dung-removal machines can be used to save time and labour; in dairy goat farming, the animals are milked in an adjacent milking parlour. The goats are fed from outside the pen using mangers or troughs; each animal must have sufficient space at the trough. The group size per pen should be around 20 to 30 (max. 40) animals to ensure proper supervision. Freezing temperatures are not harmful because the animals are able to move around.

Pasturing and paddock keeping

This method of husbandry demands a special alertness to the lively nature of goats. Weak spots in fences, netting or mesh will be exploited and used as escape routes. Despite their modest needs in terms of food, goats are very picky animals and prefer delicacies such as clover and herbs. Searching for these leads to a lot of moving around and feed substitution. A good option for pasture fences is permanent fencing with posts and wire (around 120 cm high) or electric knotted mesh fencing, which is easy to set up and move so that strip grazing can be introduced. A good supply of water at pasture is crucial; in summer, plenty of shade (field shelters, trees) should be available.

Another method of pasturing, but one which is heavily discouraged in the UK, is

staking. In this method, each goat is tethered to a long chain staked into the ground, allowing it to graze the grass around the stake. Close supervision is essential because the goats have limited freedom of movement and are defenceless against threats such as dogs.

Herded flocks of goats have recently made a return to Germany as part of landscape conservation projects. They can also be found in some Alpine and Mediterranean countries. Accompanied by a shepherd, the goats go out to pasture in the mornings and return in the evenings.

Individual goats are often kept **with other animals**. Shepherds use goats as foster mothers for orphaned lambs, while some horse owners keep a single goat as a companion for their horse or pony.

2

Sick sheep and goats

Before describing each disease in detail, we start by explaining a number of basic terms used in veterinary medicine.

The concept of disease (health, environment, disease resistance)

For an animal to be healthy, its body and organs need to function without disruption. **Disease** is the result of a disruption of normal physiological functions. How and whether a disease develops depends on the animal's overall condition (**constitution**), its susceptibility to disease (**predisposition**) and the effects of external and internal **causes of disease** (e.g. pathogens, environmental factors, metabolic disorders). A pathogen is anything that causes a disease, including viruses, bacteria, fungal organisms and parasites. Sheep and goats are especially prone to parasite infestation.

Detection of disease, health monitoring

Disease in an animal manifests via **signs** (**symptoms**) which can be subtle or pronounced. They include fever, diarrhoea (scours), coughing, poor appetite and inability to stand ('downer animals'). Based on the symptoms, a thorough examination of the animal, and tests on materials such as blood, dung and urine, it is possible to identify the disease (**diagnosis**). Treatment (**therapy**) depends on the diagnosis, which also allows a prediction to be made regarding the future course of the disease (**prognosis**).

In order to identify a disease, however, it is important to know what constitutes normal behaviour in a healthy animal and to be able to recognise symptoms at an early stage. The more you know about normal behaviour, the sooner you will spot anything abnormal. Early detection of symptoms, accurate diagnosis and prompt treatment improve the prospects of recovery for the animal concerned and help to protect the remainder of the flock.

The following are therefore vital:

- close observation and monitoring of animals,
- correct assessment of symptoms, no 'waiting and seeing',
- diagnosis and treatment by a veterinary surgeon.

Disease prevention

All of the measures outlined below are designed to prevent diseases from developing. They do not offer 100% protection but they do help to shorten the duration of a disease and to reduce its severity. Good physiological resilience (**resistance**), which plays a vital role in defending against infectious disease, can develop only if animals are kept in welfare-friendly conditions and fed a healthy diet.

Feeding and husbandry

A balanced diet geared to performance levels and specifically tailored to ruminants is the key foundation stone for any sheep or goat keeping operation. Poor-quality or spoiled feed, a lack of certain nutrients (e.g. minerals, trace elements), and feed containing toxic plants lead to deficiency diseases, metabolic disorders and poisoning. They also increase an animal's susceptibility to infectious disease by impairing the body's natural defences.

Welfare-friendly husbandry also helps to strengthen the immune system. Conversely, poor air quality in buildings encourages pneumonia and other respiratory diseases. Dry bedding, good ventilation and enough space for every animal, including space at the feed trough, are basic prerequisites for indoor farming. In summer, animals should be able to find shade or shelter.

Every sheep or goat keeper should create the best possible conditions for their animals. Your veterinary surgeon will be pleased to help.

General measures: care, disinfection

Care includes:

- hoof care, foot baths,
- inspecting pastures (removing toxic plants, draining boggy areas),
- prompt shearing including treatment for ectoparasites,
- after long spells of rain in hot weather, checking damp spots in the fleece for maggots.

Disinfection is used to target and eliminate undesirable micro-organisms, either during the course of a disease (to reduce pathogen numbers) or as a purely preventive measure (to minimise the pressure of infection, e.g. in buildings). Suitable disinfectants have been tested by the German Veterinary Medical Society (DVG) and are published in its latest list of disinfectants (currently List 13) and in the UK see DEFRA website. Your veterinary surgeon can provide you with relevant information. When choosing a disinfectant, check whether it is approved for use in **occupied** or **unoccupied buildings** (irritation of the lining of the nose promotes respiratory disease).

Coccidia parasites cannot be controlled with conventional farm disinfectants. Special disinfectants are available to control the eggs and oocysts of this parasite.

Specific measures: vaccination, medication

Vaccination is used to prevent specific infectious diseases. Vaccines stimulate sheep and goats to produce their own antibodies, equipping them to deal with the pathogens concerned. Vaccination either prevents infection or reduces the severity of the disease (active immunisation).

Farmers can vaccinate their own stock as long as they are suitably trained and the vaccines are supplied in accordance with the Veterinary Medicines Regulations.

Vaccines for farm animals fall into two categories, namely POM-VPS and POM-V:

- POM-VPS (Prescription-Only Medicine – Veterinarian, Pharmacist, Suitably Qualified Person). This is a medicine for food-producing animals, which must be prescribed by a veterinarian, pharmacist, or SQP (either orally or in writing) and which must be supplied by one of those groups of people in accordance with the prescription.
- POM-V (Prescription-Only Medicine – Veterinarian). A medicine that must be prescribed (either orally or in writing) by a veterinarian to animals under his care following a clinical assessment, and which may be supplied by a veterinarian or pharmacist in accordance with the prescription.

The vaccines licensed for use in sheep and goats are listed in the table opposite.

Flock-specific vaccines against Salmonellae, Pasteurellae, Orf and Chlamydial abortion are manufactured by specialised laboratories or pharmaceutical firms. Johne's disease vaccines have been used for years in the UK.

The basic principle when it comes to veterinary drugs is that they should be used as little as possible but as much as necessary. Medication use should be targeted and based on accurate diagnosis. This requires good cooperation between animal keeper and veterinary surgeon.

As a top priority, sheep and goat keepers should devise a worming programme tailored to the method of husbandry, local conditions and the parasite burden of the flock or herd.

Preventing losses of lambs

The following diseases should be considered and appropriate action taken:

- **enzootic abortion:** vaccination of dams, emergency vaccination (flock-specific vaccination),
- **navel infection:** disinfection with iodine,
- **Orf:** flock-specific vaccination,
- **poor colostrum intake:** newborns need to receive sufficient colostrum, using frozen or freeze dried supplies if necessary,
- **mastitis in dams:** mastitis (inflammation of the udder) in the dam deprives the lambs of milk, which can be remedied by supplementary feeding with milk replacer; treatment,
- **diarrhoeal diseases:** identify and treat the cause,
- **Enterotoxaemia (pulpy kidney disease):** preventive vaccination of ewes, vaccination of lambs from week 2 after birth.

Avoiding the introduction of pathogens

Every animal coming into a flock from outside brings a risk of introducing pathogens (viruses, bacteria, parasites).

Keeping new animals under **quarantine** – isolated from the others in a completely separate building with dedicated tools and equipment – substantially reduces this risk. Quarantine should last for at least 2–3 weeks, ideally longer. Animals should be observed closely during this time. Faecal testing, and possibly blood tests, should be carried out.

Selected vaccines used in sheep and goats.

Disease	*Commercial name of vaccine*	*Administration (Refer to manufacturer's data sheet) (MA = Marketing Authorisation (UK))*
Foot rot	Footvax	No MA for use in goats. Must be used as part of comprehensive foot rot control strategy.
Clostridial diseases	Bravoxin (10 in 1)	No MA for use in goats.
	Covexin 8 (8 in 1)	No MA for use in goats.
	Covexin 10 (10 in 1)	No MA for use in goats.
	Lambivac (4 in 1)	No MA for use in goats. This vaccine is widely used in the UK goat sector to control enterotoxaemia under cascade principles. Field evidence suggests that after an initial priming and secondary dosing (as per the sheep datasheet), boosters should be administered at least **every 3 months**.
Pasteurellosis	Ovipast plus	No MA for use in goats.
Combined Clostridial and Pasteurella infection.	Heptavac P plus	No MA for use in goats.
	Ovivac P plus	No MA for use in goats.
Enzootic abortion (EAE) – *Chlamydophila* abortion.	CEVAC Chlamydia	No MA for use in goats.
	Mydiavac	No MA for use in goats.
	Enzovax	No MA for use in goats.
Johne's disease	Gudair	MA for both sheep and goats in the UK.
Louping ill	Louping ill vaccine	No MA for use in goats.
Schmallenberg virus	SBVvax	No MA for use in goats.
Orf (contagious pustular dermatitis)	Scabivax forte	No MA for use in goats.
Toxoplasma abortion	Toxovax	No MA for use in goats.
Bluetongue serotype 8	Zulvac 8 Ovis	No MA for use in goats.
Q Fever	Coxevac	MA for goats, but No MA for use in sheep.

Full information on each vaccine including administration routes, frequency of boosters, contra-indications in the UK at NOAH (National Office of Animal Health), website: http://www.noahcompendium.co.uk/Compendium-datasheets_A-Z/Datasheets/-23637.html

New arrivals should be monitored for the following in particular:

- respiratory diseases,
- foot rot,
- drug-resistant parasites,
- Orf,
- enzootic abortion,
- Maedi-visna/CAE.

3

Tips on identifying diseases

Close monitoring of your sheep and goats helps you to spot departures from the norm, which then require further investigation. Unusual observations should always be reported to your veterinary surgeon.

Movements

Lethargy, disorientation, unsteady or wide-legged gait, circling, head drooping, 'downer' animals, repeated lying down and standing up, kicking limbs or head tilt point to nervous system disease, metabolic disorders, poisoning or mastitis.

Breathing

In a healthy animal, the respiratory rate is 12 to 25 breaths per minute. The figure is higher in younger animals and at higher ambient temperatures. An increased respiratory rate with an abdominal component (heaving flanks) is a sign of pneumonia.

Fever

Temperatures are taken rectally. Normal body temperature is 38.5 to 39.5°C. Exercise and heat produce a rise in temperature that can be characterised as normal. Fever occurs in systemic infections caused by viruses or bacteria, but also in cases of mastitis or metritis.

Head

The mucous membranes of the nose, mouth and eyes should be pale pink in colour. Membranes that are whitish, yellowish or too pale may be caused by a circulatory disorder, jaundice, or blood loss due to a parasite infestation. A swelling under the jaw can be a sign of a heavy worm burden.

Lungs

When examining the airways, listen for sounds such as rattling, whistling, snoring or coughing, and look for nasal discharge, which may be watery, whitish, thick or runny. These clues may point to the presence of pasteurellosis or pulmonary adenomatosis (jaagsiekte).

Rumen

Behind the ribs on the left side of the body lies the rumen. The regular expansions and contractions of this organ are visible and can be felt by placing a hand on the animal's flank. Rumination ('chewing the cud') also provides information about rumen activity. Digestive disorders impair the function of the rumen and can therefore alter an animal's cud-chewing behaviour.

Udder

Noticeable behavioural changes in female animals should prompt an examination of the udder. Depending on how full the udder is, it may be soft to firm but it should not be lumpy, painful or hot to the touch. Changes in the udder may indicate mastitis.

Hindquarters

Diarrhoeal diseases (scours) invariably lead to severe soiling of the hindquarters and tail area. Diarrhoea has multiple causes, so a diagnosis is essential. In warmer conditions, soiling attracts flies, which then lay their eggs, leading to maggot infestation or 'fly strike'.

Hooves and joints

Lameness can be caused by hoof diseases and inflamed joints (arthritis). Foot rot and bacterial conditions due to infected navels in lambs require further investigation to identify the cause.

Fleece, coat

Itching, rubbing and loose strands of wool are signs of mange or a fungal infection. This requires thorough investigation for the presence of external parasites, including mites. As part of mange diagnosis, the veterinary surgeon will take a skin scraping for examination.

Overestimating your own skill at detecting and identifying diseases can lead to unnecessary losses of animals. If in doubt, always consult your veterinary surgeon. The keeper's own checks and findings will help the vet to establish a diagnosis and initiate treatment.

Disease prevention programme

Interval between weaning and the next service

Dams

- Dry dams off by moving them to leaner pastures or cutting feed rations; do not reduce their supply of drinking water!
- allow dams to recover: leave at least eight weeks between lambing and the next service;
- select dams for further breeding;
- check for foot rot; treat or vaccinate if necessary;
- vaccinate against pulpy kidney disease if the flock is at particular risk;
- vaccinate against pasteurellosis regardless of whether there is a particular risk or not;
- investigate and treat for worms;
- treat for ectoparasites;
- around three weeks before service, increase the dams' level of feeding ('flushing') to stimulate oestrus and improve lambing results.

Weanlings

- If no worm-free pastures are available, monitor levels of worm infestation by testing; treat with suitable wormers;
- select female lambs for breeding and include in the pulpy kidney and pasteurellosis vaccination programme.

Rams

- Assess breeding rams carefully; cull under-performers and those with poor conformation;
- make sure you have enough rams for the number of ewes to be served; quarantine bought-in rams and blood-test them, e.g. for maedi-visna;

- check for foot rot;
- vaccinate against pulpy kidney, pasteurellosis and foot rot.

Interval between service and early pregnancy

Dams

- Provide a good supply of food and minerals;
- avoid stress and unnecessary treatments or interventions;
- treat for liver fluke if necessary.

Rams

- Monitor closely and offer plenty of food to avoid weight loss during the mating season;
- observe rams closely during mating to spot poor performance.

Interval until the end of pregnancy

Dams

- Identify dams which have lost weight and establish the cause;
- do not feed poor-quality silage (listeriosis) or poor-quality hay (abortion);
- conduct blood tests to identify deficiencies (minerals);
- check for foot rot;
- check for ectoparasites;
- if necessary, treat for worms in the final third of pregnancy using a suitable wormer;
- treat for liver fluke if necessary;
- increase level of feeding, starting around eight weeks before lambing;
- vaccinate against pulpy kidney and pasteurellosis;
- have all premature births investigated by a laboratory.

Lambing time

- All dams having problems during pregnancy or lambing (e.g. vaginal prolapse, mastitis, pregnancy toxaemia, dystocia) should be marked;
- all dams receiving lambing assistance should be treated with antibiotics (by your veterinary surgeon);
- monitor the dams' milk yield;
- get supplies of colostrum ready for the lambs;
- mark, monitor and observe suspect, sickly lambs. If necessary, isolate them so they can be cared for and reared separately;
- disinfect navels with iodine;
- if necessary, give the dams a magnesium supplement to prevent grass tetany;
- treat the dams for worms if necessary;
- treat the lambs for coccidiosis if necessary;
- vaccinate the lambs against pulpy kidney and pasteurellosis at 2–3 weeks old if they are at risk;
- treat for liver fluke in at-risk regions.

Herding dogs

- Treat dogs with effective products to control roundworms and tapeworms.

4

Medicine cabinet

Stock a medicine cabinet with the help of your veterinary surgeon. Be sure to comply with the regulations governing the acquisition, storage and use of veterinary drugs.

- **Prescription-only medicines** are available solely through your veterinary surgeon or from a pharmacy (on veterinary prescription);
- **over-the-counter medicines** can be obtained from your veterinary surgeon and/or from a pharmacy;
- **freely available medicines** are sold by agricultural retailers, chemists, veterinary surgeries and pharmacies.

Key equipment and materials

Every medicine cabinet should contain the following:

- thermometer,
- hoof knife,
- obstetric rope,
- disposable plastic syringes for giving medication in liquid form (5 ml, 20 ml capacity),
- stomach tube with funnel (for lamb rearing),
- baby bottle with rubber teat.

Handling medication

Medicines for use in animals should be stored in a cool, dry place out of the reach of children and unauthorised persons. When stocking your medicine cabinet, always note the expiry dates. Medicines that are out of date are less effective and may cause harmful side effects. When using veterinary medicines, you must comply with the **withdrawal periods** for milk, meat and internal organs. Your veterinary surgeon will inform you of these and they can also be found in the package insert.

Any erratic, unplanned or experimental use of medicines should be avoided!

Wormers and external parasite treatments (dips, sprays, pour-ons, etc.) should be used only as required. Antibiotics should be given as directed by your veterinary surgeon (dose, duration, etc.).

5

UK laws governing sheep and goat keeping

The most important laws concern the duty to notify or report the diseases listed below and the regulations on the usability of carcasses.

A duty to notify the Animal and Plant Health Agency (APHA) applies to veterinary surgeons and any person in charge of animals. Notifiable diseases of sheep and goats in some parts or all of the UK are:

- Aujeszky's disease,
- brucellosis,
- foot-and-mouth disease,
- Anthrax,
- peste des petits ruminants*,
- sheep pox and goat pox*,
- blackleg,
- rabies,
- scrapie,
- bluetongue,
- contagious agalactia,
- contagious epididymitis,
- epizootic haemorrhagic disease,
- Rift Valley fever,
- sheep scab,
- vesicular stomatitis.

* NB: Not currently present in Central Europe

Carcasses of sheep and goats with the following are **unfit** for human consumption:

- Emaciation,
- Presence of larval cestodes,
- jaundice,
- listeriosis,
- salmonellosis,
- tetanus,
- tuberculosis,
- wetness (i.e. PSE meat),
- other general disorders,
- absence of slaughter and meat inspection,
- presence of veterinary drug residues.

In the UK the situation is as follows. A more complete source of these regulations can be found in the UK Government website, under Sheep and Goats: Welfare Regulations. They apply in many other regions but readers should check their local government website for latest advice.

The welfare of sheep is protected by the Animal Welfare Act 2006, under which it is an offence to cause unnecessary suffering to any animal. The Act also contains a Duty of Care to animals – this means that anyone responsible for an animal must take reasonable steps to make sure the animal's needs are met. It must be ensured that animals are free from hunger, thirst, discomfort, pain, injury and disease. Animals should not suffer fear or distress and should be free to express their normal behaviour.

- **Cross Compliance, good practice and duty of care**: general welfare requirements for all farmed animals – including sheep and goats – are outlined in the Welfare of Farmed Animals (England) Regulations 2007.
- **Housing, shelter and environment**: fences and hedges need to be well maintained to prevent injury to the animals. For animals not kept in buildings, some sort of shelter should be provided where necessary.
- **Feeding and watering**: equipment needs to be designed and sited to minimise contamination or freezing. Diet must be balanced and adequate to maintain full health and vigour. Statutory Management Requirement 11 sets out the Cross Compliance obligations regarding food and feed law for livestock.
- **Stock keeping and milking**: anyone attending to farm animals must be familiar with the welfare code for the species.
- **Breeding and pregnancy**: any natural or artificial breeding procedures that may cause suffering or injury to animals shouldn't be used, except where this is momentary or not likely to cause lasting injury.
- **Welfare during transportation, at market and at shows**: When moving animals, they must be transported in a way that won't cause them injury or unnecessary suffering.
- **Welfare at slaughter and fallen stock**: The welfare of animals at the time of slaughter or killing is covered by European Union Directive 93/119 and UK regulations. Carcasses awaiting collection MUST be covered and protected from dogs, other wild mammals and birds.

6

Laboratory testing options for sheep and goat keepers

Whole carcasses, organs and other materials (e.g. swabs, blood samples) can be submitted for laboratory investigation. Contact your veterinary surgeon for details on the samples required and submission to your local laboratory.

Carcasses (post mortem)

Dead animals should be submitted for investigation immediately, before decay sets in, in order to establish the cause of disease or death and to prevent further animal losses. Appropriate flock or herd treatment can be initiated once the cause has been ascertained.

Whole organs, parts of organs, foetal material with afterbirth

Diseases can be identified by investigating lesions such as organ changes noticed during slaughter. In addition to epidemic abortions, there are also non-contagious causes of abortion. Investigation can help to clarify the cause.

Dung samples (parasitology, bacteriology, virology)

Diarrhoeal diseases often have an infective cause (parasites, bacteria, viruses), which can be detected by appropriate investigation. Samples should be collected using a plastic glove, either directly from the rectum or from a pile of fresh dung.

Samples must be submitted in clearly labelled, tightly sealed plastic containers. Paper and glass containers are not suitable.

Milk samples (bacteriology, serology)

Regular bacteriological testing of milk is essential for all dairy operators selling milk from sheep or goats or using milk to make cheese. Apart from identifying pathogens that can infect humans, testing also detects mastitis agents; targeted treatment can then be initiated on the basis of antibiotic sensitivity testing.

Milk testing can also detect antibodies to maedi-visna infection in sheep, CAE in goats and Q fever in both. Availability of testing differs between countries. In the UK testing for CAE and Johne's disease is offered commercially in milking goats, but individual tests are not available.

Milk samples for testing should be submitted in clearly labelled, clean and sterile plastic containers. The skin of the teat should be cleaned and disinfected thoroughly before taking samples.

External parasites (microscopy)

Parasites are collected carefully from the coat and fleece and submitted in a screw-topped container. In cases of mange mite infestation, a skin scraping is taken from the margins of a lesion and submitted in a clean plastic container.

Blood samples

Blood samples are taken by the veterinary surgeon and tested in the laboratory according to his or her instructions.

Sending samples

All materials submitted for investigation must be fresh and kept refrigerated. They should be transported or dispatched to the laboratory in tightly sealed, unbreakable containers.

Carcasses, organs and foetal material should be taken directly to the laboratory. Persons arriving with samples should be familiar with the farm or flock. They should either bring a veterinary surgeon's report with them or be able to describe the disease situation themselves.

7

Harmful substances and feed poisoning

Nitrate/nitrite poisoning

Main symptoms

- *Restlessness*
- *Increased pulse and respiratory rate*
- *Collapse*

General: Nitrates accumulate in fodder plants, especially those grown using nitrogenous fertilisers. Fodder plants with special nitrate-storing properties – such as maize, beet leaves, and fresh, growing cereals – can contain more than 1% nitrate. When sheep and goats eat large amounts of such feed, micro-organisms ('rumen micro-flora') in their gut convert the nitrate into toxic nitrite. The toxic effects of nitrate/nitrite also depend on the levels of dry matter, readily soluble carbohydrate and vitamin C in the feed, and on the rumen pH. Once accustomed to such feed, sheep will tolerate up to 6% of their nitrogen needs in the form of nitrate.

Symptoms: The symptoms of acute poisoning are movement disorders, restlessness, faster pulse, higher respiratory rate, collapse and coma.

Diagnosis: The diagnosis is often based on the local conditions, e.g. grazing on newly fertilised pastures, animals escaping and eating fresh, growing cereals.

Treatment: In acute cases, treatment is usually unsuccessful. Treatment is given by the vet in the form of 4% methylene blue in sugar solution, administered intravenously.

Preventive measures: Animals should be prevented from eating fresh, growing cereals. Feeds with a high nitrate content should be avoided. Pastures treated with a nitrogenous fertiliser should not be grazed until after the product has been rained in.

Photosensitivity

Main symptoms

- *Reddening of exposed skin*
- *Itching*
- *Blisters*

General: There are two types of photosensitivity: primary and secondary. Cases of unknown origin are also seen. In primary photosensitivity, the ingestion of certain substances (plants, medication) produces inflammation of the skin on exposure to sunlight. Secondary photosensitivity is generally the result of liver damage caused by certain compounds found in plants. Skin disease follows due to the poor metabolic performance of the damaged liver.

Primary photosensitivity: Directly photosensitising compounds are found in buckwheat (not widely grown) and St John's Wort. These compounds alter the skin cells with the result that they react to sunlight in the same way as to sunburn. Some wormers (e.g. phenothiazine) have a similar effect.

Secondary photosensitivity: This liver-related form of photosensitivity is caused by animals ingesting harmful substances that attack the liver. The affected liver is unable to break down all of the plant compounds, with the result that photosensitising substances build up in the skin. When activated by sunlight, these substances destroy the skin cells.

Photosensitivity of unknown origin: The mechanism behind sensitivity to light after eating certain plants remains unexplained. Plants responsible include lucerne, red clover, vetches, rapeseed and smartweeds.

Symptoms: The first sign is a reddening of exposed bare skin on the head and ears. Other areas not protected by coat or wool are also affected as the condition progresses. The reddened skin is very itchy, causing animals to scratch and rub. As in cases of sunburn, animals can develop blisters followed by skin inflammation.

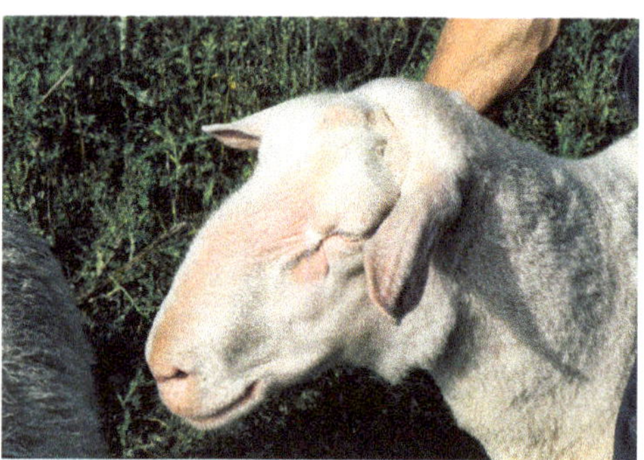

Photosensitivity: reddening of exposed skin on the ears and muzzle

Treatment and preventive measures: Once an accurate diagnosis has been made, affected animals should be moved indoors or to a shady pasture. It takes a while for the photosensitising substances in the skin to break down, so the condition can recur on exposure to sunlight even after the original symptoms have subsided. Treatment is necessary only in cases of serious skin inflammation. Animals should not be grazed on pastures containing St John's Wort or other plants that may cause photosensitivity.

Moulds in feed

General: Certain types of mould produce metabolic substances that are harmful to health. Known as **mycotoxins**, they are produced by storage moulds such as *Aspergillus* and *Penicillium*. Other moulds (*Fusarium* = field fungus) attack and damage plants such as maize and cereals. They also produce toxins (*Fusarium* toxins include zearalenone and trichothecene) that are harmful to human and animal health.

Preventive measures: Feed clean, mould-free feedstuffs. If in doubt, avoid using the feed and have it checked by a research institute or approved laboratory. Treatment can be attempted but generally has a poor chance of success.

The main mycotoxin diseases in sheep and goats.

Origin	Toxin	Symptoms
Field fungus (*Fusarium*)	Trichothecene	Feed refusal, isolation, salivation, nasal discharge, staggering gait, diarrhoea
	Zearalenone	Partly broken down in the rumen, so no special importance
Storage moulds	Aflatoxins	Reduced performance, runts, weakened immune system
	Ochratoxins*	Kidney damage, frequent urination, increased water intake

*Sheep are less sensitive than other species.

Plant poisoning

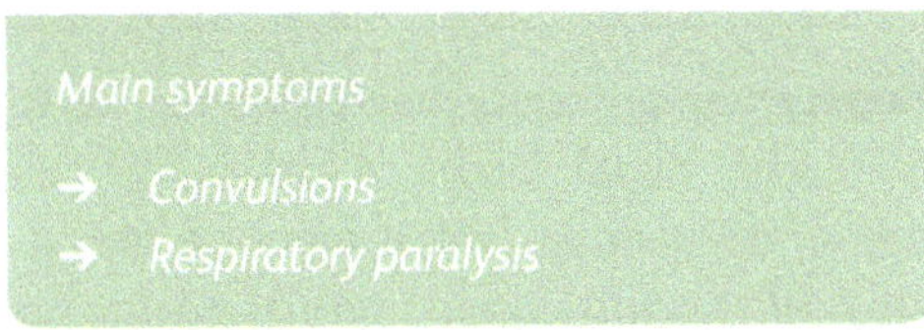

General: Plant poisoning is a rare occurrence, as sheep will avoid harmful plants if they have enough food and access to pasture. But it does happen, either due to thoughtless behaviour by gardeners or lack of knowledge on the part of sheep keepers. Every keeper should therefore be able to identify certain poisonous plants. Special attention should be paid to toxic garden plants and ornamentals, as these are often dumped on pasture land, where sheep can gain access to them. Particularly important are **yew** *(Taxus baccata),* **juniper** *(Juniperus sabina),* **white cedar** *(Thuja occidentalis),* **rhododendron** (*Rhododendron* sp.) and **ragwort** *(Seneco jacobaea).*

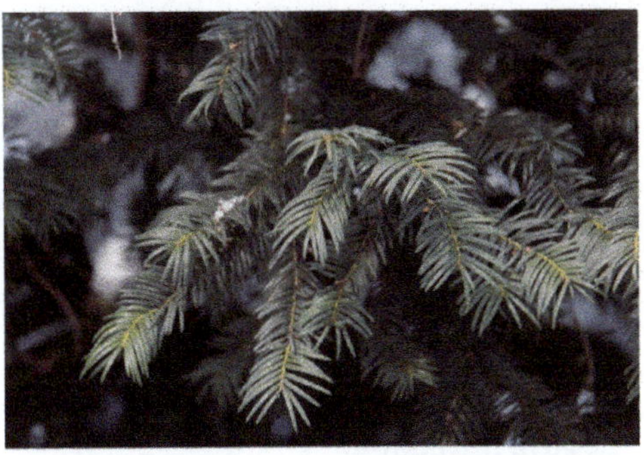

Yew *(Taxus baccata)*

Symptoms:

- **Yew poisoning.** Sheep and goats eat the branches, which contain large amounts of the toxin. Around 10 g of yew branches per kg of body weight (BW) can prove fatal for sheep. Yew poisoning is peracute, i.e. the toxins enter the bloodstream quickly, leading to respiratory and cardiac paralysis. Treatment invariably comes too late.
- **Juniper poisoning.** Juniper tips are toxic to ruminants. The toxin causes inflammation. Animals show convulsions and die due to respiratory paralysis.
- **White cedar poisoning.** The scale-like leaves of this plant contain toxins that cause inflammation and convulsions.
- **Rhododendron poisoning.** This ornamental plant contains a toxin to which sheep and goats are especially sensitive. The toxin causes inflammation, central nervous system excitation, respiratory paralysis and rumen regurgitation, which is the most common and consistent feature in the UK.
- **Ragwort poisoning.** Symptoms range from a lack of energy and general malaise through to liver damage.

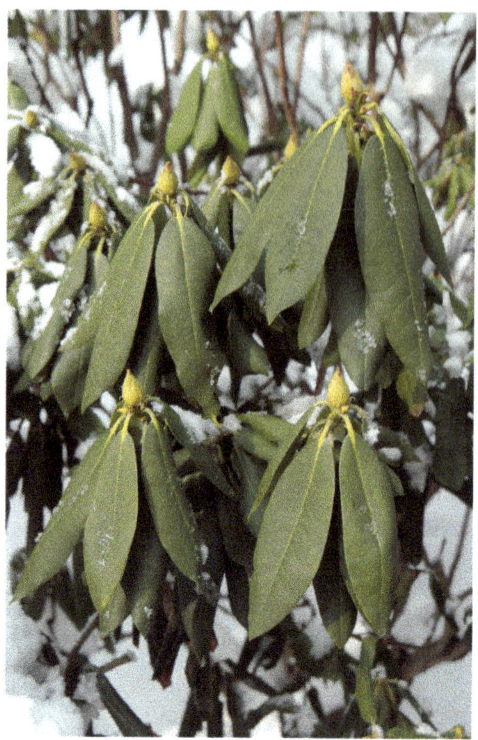

Rhododendron sp

Treatment: Poisoning is always treated according to the symptoms. However, treatment is non-specific and often unsatisfactory.

Preventive measures: Animals should be prevented from eating toxic plants. It is important to inspect pastures regularly and to have a good knowledge of toxic plants. If in doubt, contact your local research institute or plant protection service and have the plants in question tested.

Heavy metal poisoning

General: The toxic heavy metals that pose a risk to sheep and goats include lead and copper. Cases of cadmium, mercury or arsenic poisoning tend to be rare. Poisoning risks for animals result either from the ingestion of heavy metals near industrial sites such as leadworks or mines, or from the use of heavy metals such as copper in mineral mixes.

Copper poisoning

Main symptoms

- *Acute: diarrhoea, haematuria, convulsions, anaemia*
- *Chronic: weight loss, jaundice, haematuria, eczema*

General: Sheep are especially sensitive to this heavy metal. Doses as low as 10 to 20 mg/kg BW can be fatal if ingested repeatedly. Feed containing more than 15 mg of copper per kg of dry matter has a toxic effect. Sheep-milk replacer containing more than 30 mg of copper per kg BW will cause chronic copper poisoning, and 1 g of copper per day can be fatal for heavily pregnant sheep.

- **Symptoms of acute poisoning:** Diarrhoea, haematuria (blood in the urine), convulsions, anaemia.
- **Symptoms of chronic poisoning:** The chronic form is most common in sheep, as mineral feeds for cattle (high copper content) are often fed to sheep as well. Symptoms of chronic copper poisoning include liver and kidney dysfunction, leading to digestive disorders, weight loss, jaundice, haematuria and eczema.
- **Treatment:** There is no treatment for chronic poisoning, as copper accumulates in body tissues and is not excreted. The primary storage organ is the liver. In cases of chronic poisoning, the liver can contain more than 400 mg of copper per kg of dry matter.
- **Preventive measures:** Make sure that the

level of copper in feed for sheep does not exceed 10 to 15 mg/kg DM.

Lead poisoning

General: Lead occurs in nature in the form of an ore (galena), which is processed (smelted), leaving gases and slag. In the past, plants growing by the side of roads with heavy traffic were often contaminated with lead. The widespread use of lead-free fuel has helped to improve this situation. Dyes containing lead, and lead pipes in old buildings, can also cause poisoning in animals. Lead paint on old doors is a common source.

Symptoms: Lead poisoning is invariably a chronic condition, leading to weight loss, reduced feed intake, anaemia, movement disorders, excitation with 'sham chewing' and signs of blindness.

Treatment: Options available to the veterinary surgeon include 'chelating' agents such as calcium sodium versenate. These agents form a complex with the lead, causing the toxic metal ions to be excreted in the animal's urine.

Preventive measures: Lead-contaminated pastures and substances containing lead should be avoided.

Feed should not contain more than 10 mg/kg DM.

Other heavy metals

As mentioned earlier, other types of metal poisoning tend to be rare and due to inattention on the part of keepers or the grazing of sheep on reclaimed industrial land.

8

Metabolic disorders and deficiency diseases

Metabolic disorders and deficiency diseases can cause serious symptoms. A balanced diet containing sufficient minerals can help to prevent these diseases.

Vitamin deficiency (vitamin A, vitamin B1)

Main symptoms

- *Movement disorders*
- *Animals lying on sides, heads stretched back*
- *Convulsions*

General: Vitamin A deficiency is rare in sheep and goats and occurs only in housed animals. Vitamin B1 (thiamine) deficiency leads to encephalomalacia (cerebrocortical necrosis = CCN) in both fattening lambs and older animals.

Vitamin A deficiency is rare in animals fed on grass, clover and lucerne as these feeds contain β-carotene, a vitamin A precursor. Maize and maize silage contain less β-carotene. The symptoms of deficiency are non-specific. Lambs fail to thrive and suffer from diarrhoea. Adult sheep become night blind and breeding rams have reduced fertility.

CCN is caused by a deficiency of thiamine (vitamin B1). Thiamine is normally produced by the rumen bacteria, but its production is disrupted if animals are fed a milk diet low in crude fibre. The uptake of thiamine from the gut can also be disrupted, e.g. in cases of diarrhoea. Feed can also contain substances that block thiamine uptake (e.g. Amprolium).

Symptoms: In the initial stages, this disease is characterised by a lack of coordination (staggering, tripping, stumbling). The animals' vision appears to be impaired. Soon, they lie on their sides with their heads stretched back, making paddling leg movements. Occasional convulsions (stiff legs) are observed. Noises and tapping on top of the skull can trigger these convulsions. Untreated animals lose consciousness and die within a week.

Treatment: In both vitamin A and vitamin B1 deficiency, the veterinary surgeon should inject the appropriate vitamin immediately. Vitamin A is injected at a dose of around 100,000 I.U. (aqueous solution), while thiamine is administered in a complex with other B vitamins (10 mg/kg BW). Treatment can be repeated after 24 hours if there is no improvement. Because CCN is hard to distinguish from grass tetany (magnesium deficiency), a solution containing magnesium can be injected subcutaneously in addition to thiamine.

Preventive measures: Sheep and goats need to receive a feed containing crude fibre in order for thiamine to be produced by the rumen bacteria. Young animals reared without their mothers can also be given vitamin A preventively once a week. However, overdosing is also toxic.

Vitamin E and selenium deficiency

Main symptoms in lambs

- *Dog-sitting posture*
- *Stiff gait*
- *Lowered head*

General: Vitamin E and selenium deficiency lead to changes in the cardiac and skeletal musculature, 'white muscle disease'.

Symptoms: Lambs may be particularly affected if their mothers are deficient. Symptoms include difficulty in standing, dog-sitting posture, a stiff, tired gait, and a lowered head.

Diagnosis: Blood tests to determine vitamin E and selenium levels.

Preventive measures: Make sure that the feed provides a regular, adequate supply of both essential additives.

Trace element deficiencies

Copper deficiency (swayback)

Main symptoms

- *Lambs: lack of stamina, ataxia, sitting like a frog*
- *Adult animals: weight loss, anaemia, brittle wool*

General: Copper deficiency occurs mainly in newborn lambs but adult animals can also be affected. Neurological symptoms are to the fore in lambs, while adult animals display anaemia, wool damage and fertility problems.

Primary copper deficiency is caused by an absolute copper deficiency on the pasture. **Secondary copper deficiency** develops despite adequate levels of copper in the feed: the copper cannot be utilised because its uptake is blocked by other substances such as molybdenum and iron. Over-liming of pastures can also cause secondary copper deficiency. Copper deficiency inhibits brain development in newborn lambs. In older lambs, it destroys nerve cells and breaks down the myelin sheath surrounding nerve fibres. Like adult animals, they also develop anaemia.

Symptoms: Newborn lambs that have not received enough copper before birth show signs of brain damage in the form of a poor suckling reflex, lack of stamina, sitting like a frog (hind limbs under the body) and general weakness.

Older lambs (a few weeks to a few months old) display buckling of the hind limbs and a 'swaying' walk (swayback). These signs are often unclear but some lambs show poor development with weight loss and a dull coat.

Copper-deficient lamb with ataxia and frog-like sitting posture

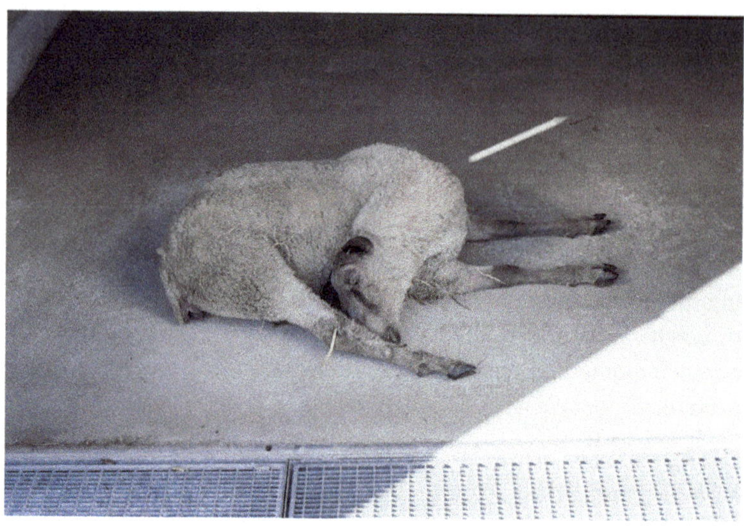

Adult animals with copper deficiency display weight loss, anaemia and brittle wool. They also have reduced fertility.

Blood tests can be carried out to detect copper deficiency. For normal levels in blood serum refer to the reference range supplied by the testing laboratory.

Treatment: Copper deficiency in newborn lambs is untreatable. Older lambs and adult sheep can be given a copper sulphate solution:

- older lambs: up to 25 ml of a 1% copper sulphate solution,
- adult sheep: up to 50 ml of a 2% copper sulphate solution.

However, treatment should be given with care because too much copper can result in copper poisoning.

Preventive measures: Mineral lick blocks containing copper should be provided. But if the exact copper content is not specified there is once again a risk of copper poisoning.

Iron deficiency

Main symptoms

- *Lambs: white mucous membranes, anaemia*

General: Iron deficiency anaemia in newborns and young animals occurs in motherless rearing and if animals are not eating enough crude fibre. Iron is an essential constituent of haemoglobin, the protein molecule in red blood cells. If there is a lack of iron in the diet (e.g. in milk-fed animals), not enough haemoglobin can be produced. This results in iron deficiency anaemia.

Other important causes of anaemia are deficiencies of the trace elements copper and cobalt. Such feed-related deficiencies should be included in the differential diagnosis of anaemia and clarified by further investigation. Sheep and goats must receive an adequate supply of these trace elements.

Symptoms: Lambs show pale mucous membranes and increased fatigue, and a greater susceptibility to other diseases. Older animals also have pale skin. A blood test gives a quick and reliable diagnosis, but other causes such as severe parasite infestation or blood loss also need to be ruled out.

Treatment: Two iron injections with an interval of 10 to 14 days produce a rapid improvement in lambs.

Preventive measures: Lambs being reared without their mothers should be given two injections of iron.

Dosage: 500 mg of iron to treat deficiency, 400 mg for prevention.

Iodine deficiency

Main symptoms

- → *Enlarged thyroid gland*
- → *Goitre*

General: Iodine deficiency occurs if the diet is lacking in iodine (**primary deficiency**) or if the processing of iodine in the thyroid gland is inhibited by certain plant constituents (e.g. in brassicas) (**secondary deficiency**). In both cases, thyroid function is disrupted. An external sign of this is a swelling of the neck known as a goitre. Iodine is essential for the functioning of the thyroid, a gland with a significant influence on the entire metabolism.

Symptoms: Iodine deficiency principally affects **unborn lambs** and **young sheep**. **Goats** are also affected. Iodine-deficient dams produce sickly or still-born lambs with a marked enlargement of the thyroid gland (goitre). Live-born lambs die shortly after birth. In iodine-deficient regions (such as the Alps), adult animals show signs of deficiency as well but goitres tend to be indistinct and there are no additional symptoms. Fertility problems have been described in such animals.

Treatment and preventive measures: Iodine deficiency can be corrected by treating with tincture of iodine (up to 0.5 ml/animal/day) for 14 days. After this, a treatment pause is required. The preventive use of mineral mixes containing iodine (0.01%) is recommended in iodine-deficient regions.

Iodine treatment is generally too late in weak newborn lambs with goitre.

Cobalt deficiency

Main symptoms

- → *Poor development of lambs*
- → *Ruffled fleece*
- → *Eating indigestible foods*

General: Cobalt is a constituent of vitamin B12, which in ruminants is produced in the rumen. A deficiency of this trace element leads to a disruption of red blood cell production. A lack of cobalt in the diet disrupts the production of vitamin B12 in the rumen. Cobalt-deficient soils are found on heaths and moorland, as well as on granite and sandstone. Fodder plants grown here do not contain enough cobalt. This lack of cobalt produces a vitamin B12 deficit in the animal, leading to anaemia due to a disruption of red blood cell production in the bone marrow.

Symptoms: Lambs fail to thrive despite good feeding and the absence of other disease. Adult animals have a ruffled fleece, eat indigestible foods such as wood, earth and bark, and drink stagnant water. The animals become progressively emaciated. A diagnosis of cobalt deficiency is confirmed in the laboratory by blood testing with a cobalt assay.

Treatment and preventive measures: Vitamin B complexes can be used to treat acute deficiency. A repeat treatment after three weeks is recommended. Cobalt is administered in the form of cobalt chloride or sulphate. Injections are ineffective. Mineral feeds should include sufficient levels of cobalt. Fertilising cobalt-deficient pastures with cobalt salts can help to prevent deficiencies.

Giving cobalt to ewes and does in late pregnancy produces a marked increase in vitamin B12 levels in their milk and prevents deficiency in the lambs and kids. At six to eight weeks old, young animals can also be given cobalt orally. This stimulates the production of vitamin B12 in the rumen.

Pregnancy toxaemia

Main symptoms in the final third of pregnancy

- ➔ *Unsteady gait*
- ➔ *Reduced feed intake*
- ➔ *Teeth grinding*
- ➔ *'Downer' animals*
- ➔ *Lack of rumen activity*

General: Pregnancy toxaemia, also known as twin lamb disease, is an often acute metabolic disorder of **pregnant sheep and goats**. It stems from a disruption of the carbohydrate and fat metabolism.

In the final stages of pregnancy, the foetuses need larger quantities of blood sugar (glucose). Especially in a multiple pregnancy, the mother's body has to supply enough glucose to ensure that the lambs have sufficient reserves in their first week of life. If the dam does not receive a good supply of easily digestible carbohydrates at this stage of pregnancy (e.g. due to incorrect feeding, crude fibre deficiency, or lack of feed), her own reserves become depleted. Her body starts to use the sugar stored in the liver and muscles. Blood sugar levels fall. Once the dam's sugar reserves are exhausted, she starts to break down body fat. This produces increasing levels of ketones, which can be detected in the blood and urine. Ketone bodies damage and paralyse the animal's nervous system.

Symptoms: The symptoms develop slowly but become increasingly apparent and almost always lead to death. The first sign is a reluctance to move. Affected animals hang back from the rest of the flock; their gait becomes stiff legged and unsteady. Their feed intake is reduced, even if good feed is available. In animals in the final stages of pregnancy, the diagnosis should be confirmed in the laboratory by testing their urine for ketone bodies. As the disease progresses, animals are seen to lie with their necks stretched out. They grind their teeth and their breathing and pulse rates are accelerated. Blood sugar levels are well below normal. Rumen activity is limited and droppings are coated with mucus. After a day or two the animals 'go down', first lying on their fronts and then on their sides. The front and hind limbs make paddling movements. The animals' breath smells fruity due to ketone bodies. Loss of consciousness is followed by death.

Treatment: Sugar levels in the blood need to be raised. To do this, the veterinary surgeon will infuse sugar solutions into the bloodstream. Sugar (dextrose) can also be given subcutaneously and may be better by this route, because when given intravenously much of it is excreted. Cortisone and vitamins are also administered, together with treatment to protect the liver. If this treatment triggers a premature birth, the animal's condition may improve spontaneously. However, treatment is often unsuccessful.

Preventive measures: In advanced pregnancy, sheep and goats need around 120 g of digestible crude protein per day. These figures are approximate guidelines, as levels of crude protein and starch units depend on the number of unborn lambs or kids. The best feed for sheep and goats is good quality, unspoiled hay, which should be provided throughout the day together with water. Supplementary feeding should consist of beet pulp, potatoes and fodder beets. Animals should also have an adequate supply of minerals, especially magnesium (licks).

Calcium and magnesium deficiency

Calcium deficiency

Main symptoms in advanced pregnancy

- → *Movement disorders*
- → *'Downer' animals with outstretched necks*

General: A drop in blood calcium levels occurs mainly in **older sheep in advanced pregnancy**; more rarely, dams are affected just after lambing. One consequence of these low calcium levels in the blood is muscular dysfunction.

In the final stages of pregnancy, unborn lambs need a lot of calcium for bone development, which has to be provided by the ewe. If the ewe is not fed enough calcium during this period, or cannot obtain enough from her bone tissue, the result is an acute calcium deficiency in the blood (hypocalcaemia). Stressors such as changes of feed, transportation or being driven for too long increase the risk of hypocalcaemia.

Symptoms: Affected sheep in late pregnancy show uncoordinated movements, reduced stamina, a swaying gait and separation from the rest of the flock. Animals then 'go down', first with their necks outstretched, and then on their sides with front legs extended. Convulsions are sometimes observed. The ears and lower parts of the limbs feel cold to the touch, even though the body temperature is usually within the normal range.

Treatment and preventive measures: The veterinary surgeon can administer calcium solutions intravenously or by subcutaneous injection (up to 80 ml). An exact diagnosis is vital to avoid confusion with pregnancy toxaemia. If a reliable diagnosis cannot be obtained, blood sugar levels should be raised prophylactically. As a preventive measure, make sure that the correct mineral supplements are being given via the feed.

Magnesium deficiency (grass tetany)

Main symptoms

- → *'Downer' animals*
- → *Convulsions*
- → *Excessive salivation*

General: A drop in levels of magnesium in the blood is called **hypomagnesaemia.** The resulting interruption of neuromuscular transmission leads to recumbency and convulsions.

The condition is observed mainly in older pregnant or lactating ewes kept on young pastures with fresh grass. Fresh, fast-growing fodder contains low levels of magnesium and its high protein content reduces the uptake of magnesium from the gut. The level of magnesium in the blood falls. A drop in outside temperatures, poor weather, transport, lactation (extra magnesium is leached out via the milk) and age are other factors which can cause a magnesium deficiency.

Symptoms: In the acute form of the disease, animals 'go down', lying on their sides with heads thrown back. Convulsions and excessive salivation are observed. Death occurs within a few hours. If the disease progresses more slowly, muscle tremors and a stiff gait are observed, and animals grind their teeth. Animals may recover from this form, but it can also progress to the acute form.

Treatment: The aim is to raise the level of magnesium in the blood. To do this, the veterinary surgeon will inject a calcium/magnesium solution intravenously. This solution should also be injected under the skin at five or six different sites, using a total dose of around 100 ml.

Preventive measures: Animals should be given a mineral mix containing sufficient magnesium oxide. If grazing fresh pastures in areas at risk of magnesium deficiency, plenty of additional roughage should be provided.

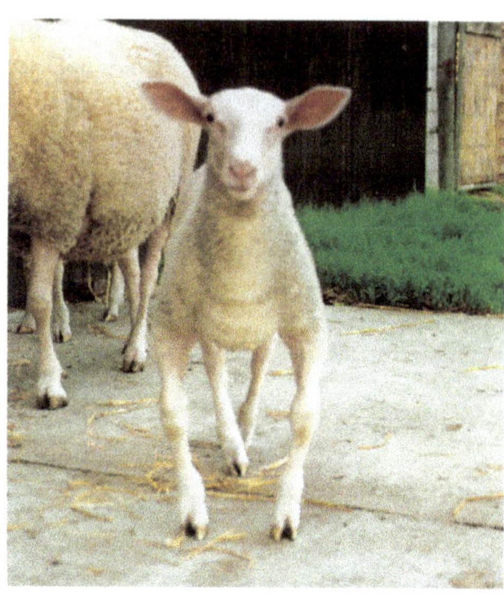

Rickets: a dairy lamb with extreme bowing of the front legs

Soft bones (rickets)

Main symptoms

- → *Deformed bones*
- → *'Bandy legs'*

General: Lack of calcium, phosphorus and vitamin D in fast-growing **lambs** housed indoors leads to leg bone deformities. Soft bones are due to an imbalance in the supply of minerals, with an abnormal calcium/phosphorus ratio and a deficiency of vitamin D.

Symptoms: Vitamin D is necessary in order to absorb sufficient calcium and phosphorus from the gut. Lambs that are deficient in vitamin D do not build up enough calcium in their bones. It is calcium that gives bones their strength. The bones and joints become thickened, especially in the growth regions at the ends of the long bones. As the lambs gain weight, their weak bones start to bend and they become bandy legged. As the disease progresses, it becomes possible to feel the thickening around the joints and at the costochondral junctions in the ventral ribcage.

Treatment: The main treatment is the giving of vitamin D (around 100 I.U.).

Preventive measures: Animals should receive a good-quality, balanced mineral feed, ideally with added vitamins. Feed wholesalers offer a wide selection.

Note: Over-dosing leads to spinal curvature and calcified organs.

Brittle bones (osteomalacia)

Main symptoms

- → *Eating unusual things*
- → *Wool eating*
- → *Tripping gait*
- → *Dull coat*

General: Brittle bones are caused by decalcification of bones in the adult animal. In the still-growing animal, a calcium/phosphorus imbalance and vitamin D deficiency lead to soft bones. In the adult animal, this deficiency causes brittle bones.

The bones of adult sheep and goats undergo a constant process of building and rebuilding, which is guaranteed only if they have a balanced supply of minerals. If a mineral feed with an incorrect calcium/phosphorus ratio is used, and if animals are kept indoors for extended periods (vitamin D deficiency), the calcium deficit is made up by leaching from the bones. As a result, the bones become brittle.

Symptoms: Animals show an increased tendency to eat unusual things (pica), or to eat wool and dirt. They develop a tripping gait and a dull coat; female animals become infertile.

Treatment and preventive measures: Vitamin D can be given orally (around 50,000 I.U.) or injected into the muscle. Take care when using oil-based solutions due to the risk of abscesses. As a long-term measure, it is important to provide sheep and goats with an adequate supply of calcium and phosphorus. The easiest way to do this is by using a mineral feed (10–20 g per day depending on age). There is no point in giving injections of calcium or phosphorus.

White muscle disease (muscular dystrophy)

Main symptoms

- *Flaccid paralysis*
- *Arched back*
- *White muscles on slaughter*

General: A lack of vitamin E and selenium in the diet leads to varying degrees of muscle tissue degeneration.

The disease can occur in newborn lambs but mainly affects **young animals**. Vitamin E and selenium deficiency occurs in regions with soils low in selenium, or where plants treated with high-sulphate fertilisers fail to take up enough selenium, or where the use of propionic acid to preserve fodder (cereals) reduces the vitamin E content.

Symptoms: In newborn lambs, the heart muscle is affected and the skeletal muscles display flaccid paralysis. The animals die of cardiac failure.

Older lambs develop well at first. As the disease takes hold, they start to arch their backs and the back muscles become stiff and painful. Their urine is darkened due to pigments produced by muscle degeneration. The heart muscle becomes affected at a later stage, leading to heart failure. When these lambs are slaughtered, the affected muscles are found to be greyish-white in colour ('white muscle').

Treatment and preventive measures: Provided that the disease is not yet advanced, a dose of selenium (around 1 mg depending on body weight) and 300 I.U. of vitamin E will produce an improvement. Treatment can be repeated after ten days. In animals that have been ill for some time and have already gone down, treatment is usually unlikely to succeed. Lambs and pregnant dams can be treated preventively with commercially available vitamin E/selenium preparations.

9

Viral infections

Infection is the process by which pathogenic agents enter, take hold of and proliferate in a host organism. An **infectious disease** is present if symptoms can be observed as a result of infection. Infectious diseases are disease processes directly related to the effects of micro-organisms (viruses, bacteria, moulds, parasites). An infectious disease is caused by:

- direct mechanical damage to organs or the whole animal;
- production (by the pathogen) of toxins which damage individual organs or the whole organism;
- metabolic changes due to the conflict between host and pathogen;
- indirect damage (e.g. reduced feed intake).

Viruses are tiny pathogens which replicate only in living cells and cause disease in plants, animals and humans. Outside a living organism, they are inactive and cannot replicate. As yet, we have very few drugs that can tackle viruses directly, so our efforts to deal with viral infections mainly involve treating the symptoms. We can help the animal's immune system in its fight against pathogens by providing good husbandry conditions and good-quality feed. Viruses can be prevented from spreading within a flock by vaccinating healthy animals or culling those with disease.

Two important new viral diseases are bluetongue and Schmallenberg virus infection.

Orf

Main symptoms

- *Lip form: pustules and scabs*
- *Foot form: pustules and reddening around the coronet*
- *Udder form: pustules and scabs*

General: Orf is a contagious viral infection of the skin around the mouth, udder and/or coronet. The mucous membranes of the mouth, oesophagus and forestomachs can also be involved. Lambs are generally worst affected. Orf can also infect humans.

Symptoms: The virus responsible for Orf (parapox virus) enters the body through minor injuries in the skin of the lips, udder and feet. After seven to ten days the typical scabs and pustules appear. Secondary bacterial infections are common. Scabs are shed after one to four weeks. Within a flock, the disease spreads through animal-to-animal contact (lambs suckle from an infected udder, then infected lambs suckle from a healthy udder). The virus can also be transmitted by equipment, artificial teats, dust and bedding. Suckling lambs and weanlings (up to ten months old) are particularly at risk.

The disease has several forms:

1. **Lip form:** A week to ten days after infection, small pustules develop around the mouth and nostrils, later merging into clusters. As the disease progresses they dry out and scab over. Large areas of skin can be covered. Depending on the severity of the lesions, affected animals can lose their appetite, leading to noticeable weight loss. In the **malignant** form, the mouth and tongue are also involved. The oesophagus and forestomachs can be affected as well. In this case, mortality is 100%.
2. **Foot form:** Pustules, reddened areas and scabs develop around the coronet and between the toes. This form of the disease is rarely observed.
3. **Mixed form:** Vesicles and pustules appear on the udder, vulva and foreskin. Healthy lambs risk becoming infected by suckling an infected udder.

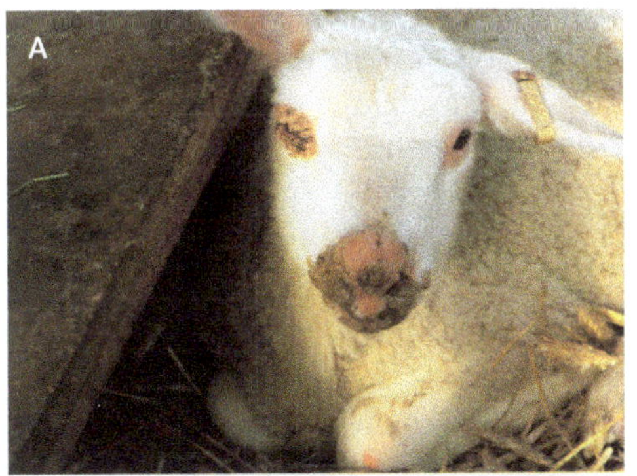

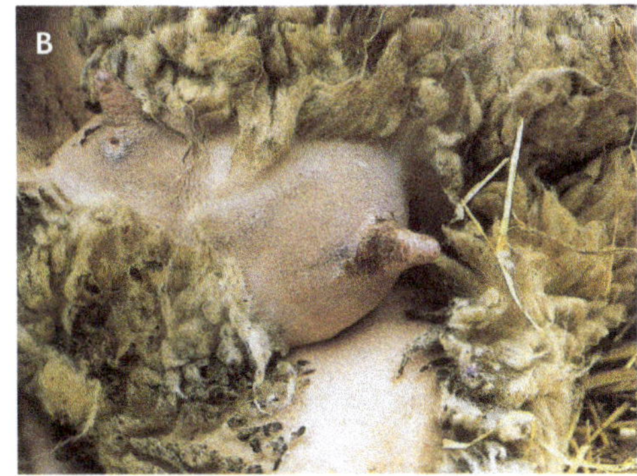

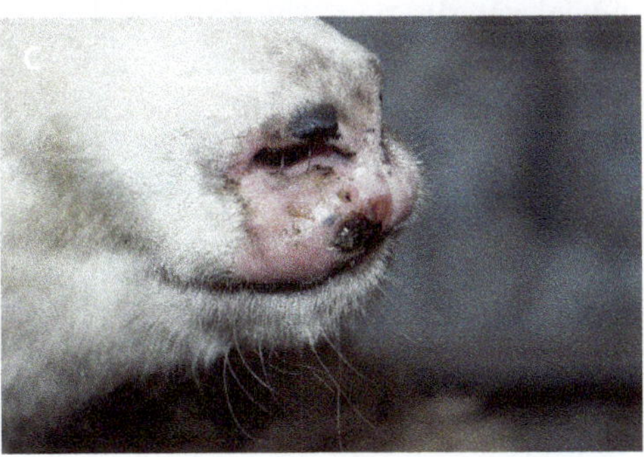

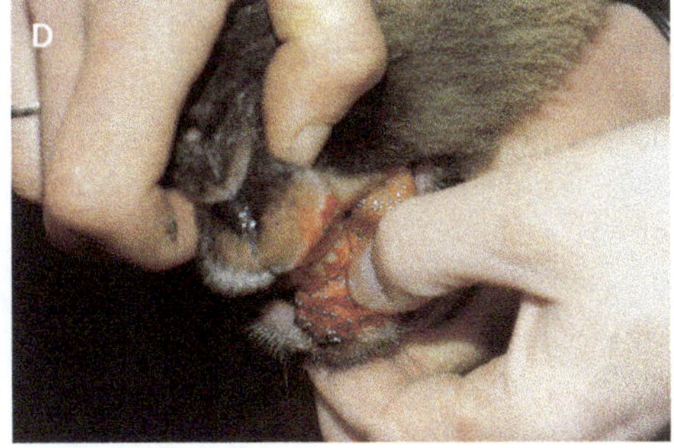

Orf: A: Orf can extend to the eyes and nostrils. B: In this form of Orf, the ewe's udder poses a risk of infection for the lambs. C: A milder form of Orf with scabbed pustules on the upper lip. D: Malignant form of Orf with involvement of mouth and gums

Once a flock has been infected, it generally has immunity for around one to two years. But this immunity does not stand up well to pressure and new lambs do not receive enough protection through their mother's milk. This means that buying in infected, asymptomatic animals can cause a fresh outbreak. The disease usually takes a milder course in **adult sheep** and in **goats**.

Treatment and preventive measures: If possible, affected animals should be isolated from the rest of the flock. Areas of skin showing lesions can be treated with antibiotic ointments, sprays or powders in order to prevent secondary bacterial infections. A vaccine for the preventive inoculation of ewes is currently available in the UK. Optimum husbandry and feed hygiene should be practised to support the body's natural defences.

Foot-and-mouth disease (FMD)

Main symptoms

- *Vesicles inside the mouth (primary vesicles)*
- *Vesicles on the feet (secondary vesicles)*

General: Foot-and-mouth disease is an acute disease of ruminants caused by various subtypes of FMD virus. In sheep, it is usually only the foot lesions that occur. In 2001, Britain suffered a devastating epidemic of FMD which also spread to France and the Netherlands and resulted in huge numbers of sheep and goats having to be killed. FMD is the subject of a state-run control programme. Sheep normally contract the disease from infected cattle. The virus enters the body through the mucous membranes of the mouth or the coronet of the hoof, where an unremarkable vesicle (primary vesicle) then develops. The virus spreads throughout the body, causing a mild fever and producing further vesicles (secondary vesicles). The vesicles form around the coronet and between the toes. Significant amounts of virus are shed throughout the period of vesicle formation and healing (lasting around ten days).

Symptoms: The first vesicles often go unnoticed. The first obvious symptom is the development of secondary vesicles on the feet, accompanied by lameness, general lethargy and reduced appetite. Three to four days after the first signs of lameness, the coronets are reddened; two days later, the appetite improves; after another three to five days, the worst is over. In lambs, the infection progresses more severely; the heart is affected and mortality can be up to 80%.

In **goats**, the disease can take either a mild or a severe form. The mouth vesicles are more obvious than in sheep, while the foot lesions are less obvious and less likely to be pronounced.

Note: FMD is a **notifiable** animal disease. All cases, even suspected ones, must be notified to the competent State Veterinary Office by the veterinary surgeon or the person in charge of the animals. All other control measures are ordered and implemented by the official veterinarian. The animals' keeper must avoid all contact with other ruminants until the official veterinarian arrives.

Rabies (Does not occur in the UK)

Main symptoms

- *Lack of appetite*
- *Anxiety*
- *Aggression*
- *Mounting*
- *Atypical movements*

General: Rabies is a viral infection of the nervous system which is transmitted by the bite of infected animals. As a rule, it affects only individual sheep or goats. The disease is fatal and also poses a significant risk to humans. It is therefore a **notifiable** disease.

Infection: The virus is transmitted by saliva from the bite of an infected animal (e.g. fox). The virus migrates along the nerve tracts to the brain. Depending on the location of the bite (i.e. distance from the head), it can take weeks for the first symptoms to appear.

Symptoms: Sheep exhibit digestive disorders, lack of appetite, anxiety and an unnaturally trusting nature ('dumb rabies'). Some animals may attack head-on. Notable symptoms are an increased sex drive, including in females (mounting other animals), restlessness, bleating and atypical movements. These are followed by paralysis with staggering and buckled limbs, drooling due to trouble swallowing, and finally animals 'go down'. The disease is invariably fatal.

Goats often display the 'dumb rabies' picture accompanied by atypical signs which progress to death.

Treatment and preventive measures: Even suspected cases of rabies are **notifiable**. All sheep keepers are alerted to the presence of the disease within a region by posting signs at the entry points to an affected town or village. Suspect animals must be confined; slaughter is prohibited. Further measures are ordered by the official veterinarian.

Note: People coming into contact with animals suspected to have rabies should be vaccinated as quickly as possible.

Scrapie

Main symptoms

- *Itching*
- *Lip smacking*
- *Trotting gait*
- *Excitability*
- *Ataxia*
- *Collapse*

General: Scrapie is a chronic, progressive disease of the nervous system which occurs in sheep and goats. Together with bovine spongiform encephalopathy (BSE), it is one of the transmissible spongiform encephalopathies (TSEs). Scrapie has existed in the UK for a long time. It was not until BSE emerged and was described in cattle that renewed attention began to be focused on scrapie in sheep and goats.

The scrapie agent is minute, smaller than a virus. Known as a **prion**, it is a simply structured but highly resilient unconventional protein that controls its own replication. Many different strains of scrapie are known; they vary in terms of clinical symptoms, pathology and biochemistry. Prions are resistant to high temperatures, light and radiation and have pH survival levels between 2.5 and 10 (i.e. they range from acidic to alkaline). They can be inactivated by autoclaving at 134 to 138°C.

Infection is transmitted via the afterbirths and amniotic fluid of infected sheep. Lambs become infected in the uterus. The buying and selling of animals spreads the agent from one flock to another and from country to country. Some sheep breeds appear to be more susceptible to the disease than others (genetic predisposition).

Four to 24 months or even as much as three years can elapse between infection and outbreak. Affected sheep are generally between two and five years old, rarely older.

Symptoms: The disease is very hard to identify in the early stages. First of all, itching is observed in individual animals. As the disease progresses, the itching increases and lip smacking and head shaking appear. Affected animals show increasing excitability and an unnatural high-stepping or 'trotting' gait. Scratching animals on the head and neck causes them to respond with nodding, head shaking and tail wagging. Excitability, tripping, erratic gait and abnormal body movements (ataxia), possibly leading to collapse, continue to increase. These symptoms do not always occur, and they do not occur in every sheep. Affected animals become debilitated and die a few weeks to six months after the onset of symptoms.

Diagnosis: The only way to obtain a reliable diagnosis in the living animal at present is to conduct an expensive **biopsy**. In the brain of a dead animal, the laboratory can perform a rapid test to detect the prions and demonstrate the typical lesions using microscopy.

Treatment and preventive measures:

Genotype	Genotype class	Risk assessment
ARR/ARR	G 1	extremely low
ARR/AHQ ARR/ ARH ARR/ARQ	G 2	low
AHQ/AHQ AHQ/ ARH AHQ/ARQ ARH/ARH ARH/ ARQ ARQ/ARQ	G 3	moderate risk
ARR/VRQ	G 4	high risk
AHQ/VRQ ARH/ VRQ ARQ/VRQ VRQ/VRQ	G 5	very high risk

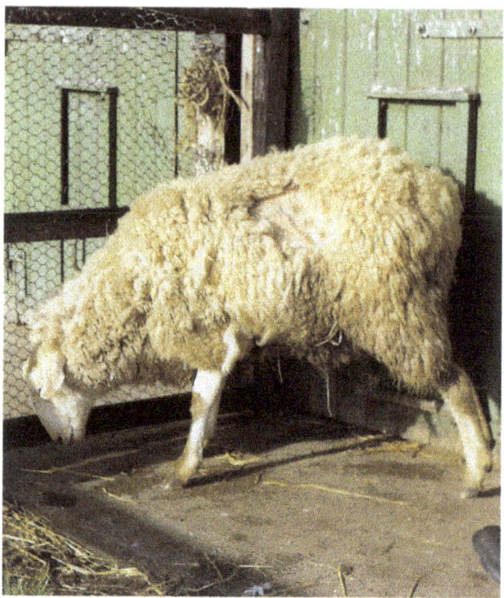

Scrapie-infected sheep showing a ruffled fleece due to scratching, and an abnormal posture

There is no treatment for TSEs. Scrapie is a **notifiable** animal disease, so all control measures are ordered by the veterinary authorities. Since a gene was found to control the production and properties of prion protein, particular arrangements of genes have been shown to alter a sheep's susceptibility to scrapie. A **genetic test** is used to examine the sheep's genetic material and, depending on the result, the sheep in question can be classed on a scale of low to high susceptibility to scrapie. The test can be carried out using an EDTA blood sample or a skin punch sample taken when inserting an ear tag.

The animals most suitable for **breeding** purposes are those in risk groups G1 and G2 with alleles ARR and AHQ. Animals in risk groups G4 and G5 should not be used for breeding (allele VRQ). When selecting breeding stock, pay particular attention to the rams to be used. All rams used for breeding should ideally belong to risk group G1. The scrapie control programme prescribed by the

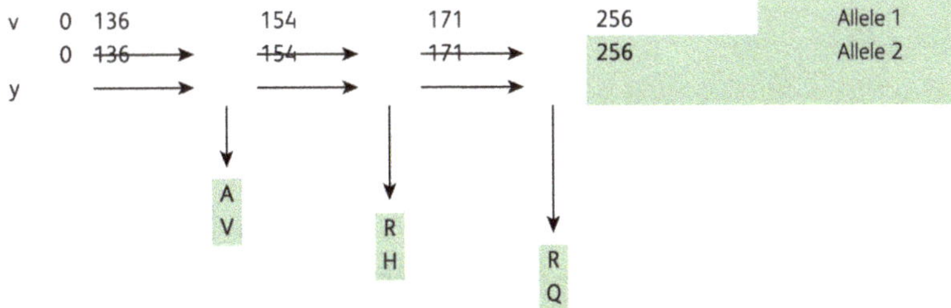

Structure of the PrP gene. Gene loci 136, 154 and 171 are crucial for susceptibility to scrapie. Scrapie susceptibility is based on a combination of 2 x 3 letters (3 on allele 1 and 3 on allele 2). A = alanine, H = histidine; Q = glutamine, V = valine, R = arginine

European Union from 2005, is based on the principle of **genotyping** and **classification into risk groups**. First, the rams are genotype and only ARR/ARR rams are accepted for breeding. In a second step, breeders should use only G1-type rams in their flocks.

Use of a designation for genotype classes of PrP alleles

Rules have been enacted in relation to sheep with particular prion protein genotypes, notably by Decision 2002/1003/EC of 18 December 2002 laying down minimum requirements for a survey of prion protein genotypes of sheep breeds and by Decision 2003/100/EC of 13 February 2003 laying down minimum requirements for the establishment of breeding programmes for resistance to transmissible spongiform encephalopathies. As specified in Annex I to Decision 2002/1003/EC, the allele is designated by a three-letter code and each genotype is designated by the combination of two alleles.

In practice, it has proved useful to agree additional designations for particular classes of genotypes.

Maedi-visna (dyspnoea/wasting)

Main symptoms

- *Rapid breathing*
- *Coughing*
- *Heaving flanks*
- *Laboured breathing*
- *Absence of fever*

General: 'Maedi' is the Icelandic word for dyspnoea or shortness of breath, which characterises one form of this viral infection, namely chronic progressive pneumonia. 'Visna' (wasting) is the form of the disease that causes central nervous symptoms. This form is rarely observed. The infection rate in a flock can range from 6 to 60%. Texels and dairy sheep are especially susceptible.

Infection: Lambs become infected in the first few days of life (perinatal infection) by drinking colostrum and milk. Airborne droplets can pass infection between animals. Direct close contact within the flock promotes transmission to older sheep. The interval between infection and outbreak can be two years or more. For this reason, symptoms are not usually expected in sheep under three years old.

Symptoms: The first symptoms are atypical: animals hang back from the rest of the

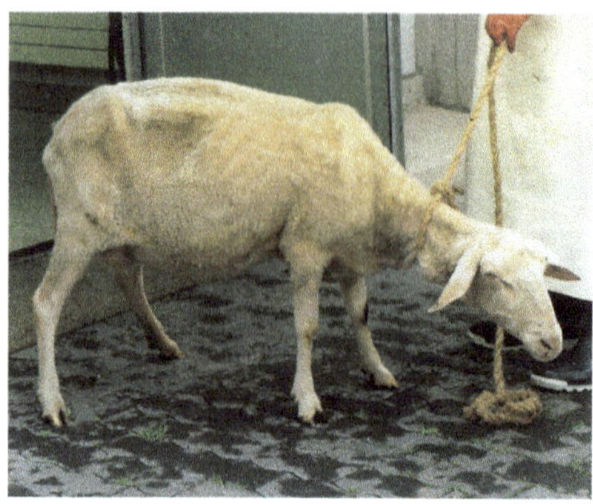

A maedi-affected sheep with severe emaciation after long-term illness

flock and appear lethargic. After stress or exertion their breathing is slightly accelerated. Occasionally a dry cough can be heard. Body temperature is normal. Unlike in other lung diseases, there is no nasal discharge. As the disease progresses, breathing becomes increasingly difficult, especially when animals are under stress. Animals start to show flared nostrils and heaving flanks; their breathing becomes laboured. The sheep lose weight despite eating normally. Severe dyspnoea and emaciation are eventually followed by death after several months.

Lambs born to affected dams are noticeably retarded in their development due to reduced milk intake. The economic losses in an infected flock can be substantial.

In the rarer, neurological form (visna), hind limb weakness is observed, becoming more marked as the disease progresses and leading to a visible sway in the hindquarters accompanied by ataxia. This change advances from hind limbs to fore limbs. Affected animals become extremely emaciated, develop severe ataxia and die after a few months.

Both maedi (respiratory form) and visna (nervous form) are invariably fatal.

Note: There is no treatment for affected animals and there are no preventive vaccinations. Maedi-visna is a **reportable** disease for veterinary surgeons, although there is no state-run control programme.

Eradication and control measures: The transmission routes of the virus (mother's milk, airborne droplets) determine the control measures: lambs must be reared without their mothers, and affected animals must be removed from the flock. For motherless rearing, it is important to monitor births in the flock closely. Newborn lambs must be separated from their mothers immediately and fed with a suitable milk replacer.

To identify potential virus shedders promptly, blood testing of all sheep in the flock is required. Testing detects positive and negative reactors. Sheep testing 'positive' are potential shedders and should be removed from the flock as quickly as possible. Further blood testing of all animals in the flock should be carried out six months later. Once again, animals testing positive are removed. A flock that has tested negative for three years in a row can be regarded as free from suspicion of maedi.

For successful eradication, these measures must be applied consistently. Motherless rearing with lambs being separated from the rest of the flock leads, in time, to the building of a maedi-free flock consisting of home-bred animals. The six-monthly blood testing of sheep with removal of 'positive' reactors will also gradually produce a maedi-free flock. However, these control measures cannot be expected to yield success in the short term.

Maedi eradication programmes have been conducted with good results by German breeding associations. Nationwide maedi eradication is practised successfully in the Netherlands.

10

Bacterial infections

Bacteria are single-celled organisms. Only a tiny proportion of all bacteria have harmful effects (i.e. are pathogenic). Bacteria are characterised by:

- a single cell with a nucleus-like structure,
- an independent metabolism,
- replication by division.

To replicate, bacteria need favourable environmental conditions, optimum temperatures (around 37°C) and an adequate supply of nutrients. These conditions are present inside the animal's body, on its mucous membranes and on its skin. Certain bacteria can also survive for several years outside an organism, i.e. in the environment.

Listeriosis

Main symptoms

- *Ataxia*
- *Circling*
- *'Downer' animals*
- *Abortions*

General: Listeriosis is an infectious disease that can cause meningitis in sheep and goats. The bacteria are generally present in the animals' environment. From there, they can infect the animal. Husbandry methods (poor ventilation, cramped conditions) can encourage the disease.

In late winter and early spring, when the sheep are indoors and feeding conditions are less than ideal, animals of any age can be affected. The source of infection is often poorly acidified silage (pH 6), which contains greater numbers of bacteria. A well-made silage has a pH of 4; Listeria is rare in such silage.

Symptoms: Apart from meningitis, the symptoms can also include abortions (in the second to fifth month of pregnancy) and stillbirths. Meningitis affects either individual animals or a group of lambs or ewes. The animals become unwell after eating grass or silage. Around 14 days after infection, animals display conjunctivitis, ataxia, circling and facial paralysis. Affected animals 'go down' and die within a week. In one- to two-week-old lambs, the infection causes diarrhoea and fever and quickly leads to death. The progression is more severe in **goats** than in sheep.

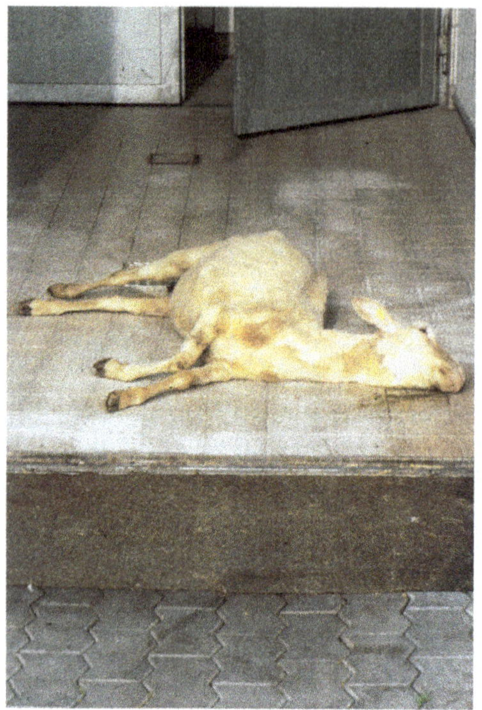

Downer sheep with outstretched neck – a typical symptom of listeriosis

Treatment and preventive measures: The main precaution is to feed good-quality silage that has been properly acidified (pH below 5). Take only the day's ration of silage from the silo; a silage face of visibly poor quality should be disposed of immediately. The feed should be changed as soon as symptoms appear. Ideally, the whole building should be emptied and disinfected. Antibiotic treatment is successful only if the disease is identified very early.

Salmonellosis

Main symptoms

- *Fever*
- *Watery, foamy diarrhoea, yellowish in lambs*

General: Salmonellosis is an infectious disease caused by various strains of **Salmonella**. In sheep and goats it can lead to diarrhoea, fever and, in extreme cases, abortion. The disease in sheep can be transmitted to humans, which makes it especially important in sheep destined for slaughter. Salmonellae are among the most common agents of animal disease worldwide and are also a major cause of zoonoses. Over 2,000 different strains of Salmonella are now known, but not all of them cause disease in humans.

Infection: Sheep and goats generally become infected by ingesting the bacteria with their feed or water. The severity of the disease depends on the numbers of bacteria ingested and on the overall health of the animal. If low numbers of pathogens are ingested and the sheep are in good overall health with strong immune defences, salmonellosis does not occur. Disease develops only in animals with a poor physical constitution. Infections with other pathogens, such as parasites, encourage outbreaks of salmonellosis.

Salmonella abortion is described elsewhere.

Symptoms: Around three to five days after infection, the animal's body temperature rises to 40–41°C. Animals seem extremely dull and have diarrhoea. The droppings are grey, loose and foamy; in lambs they are yellowish and very watery. Up to 50% of infected lambs and sheep die from this disease.

Diagnosis: Investigation of dead sheep and lambs, and possibly of dung samples, in a veterinary institute or testing facility will quickly show whether Salmonella infection is present.

Treatment and preventive measures: After antibiotic resistance testing, affected sheep are treated with a specific antibiotic. The entire course of treatment should be followed as recommended by your veterinary

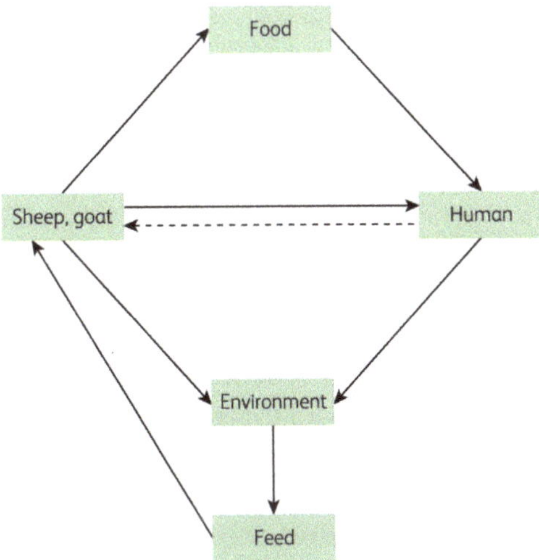

Significance of Salmonellae to humans

surgeon. Severely affected animals should be isolated from the flock, as they help to spread the pathogen. The cause of infection should be identified as quickly as possible. Potential suspects are contaminated feed, drinking water polluted with waste water, poultry (e.g. chickens, geese, ducks) and other domestic animals.

Note: Sheep keepers should be aware that they and their dogs can contract the infection from affected animals. They are therefore advised to take special care, which means paying attention to the cleaning and disinfection of equipment, feeders, troughs and clothing.

E. coli diarrhoea and septicaemia (watery mouth)

Main symptoms

- *Lethargy in first 2 to 3 days after birth*
- *Greyish-yellow diarrhoea*

General: Diarrhoea in suckling lambs in the first week of life is often caused by various pathogenic strains of *Escherichia coli.* Lambs in flocks and in housed situations tend to have a higher incidence.

An adequate supply of colostrum plays a vital role in preventing diarrhoeal diseases in the first week of life. Adult sheep have developed immunity to pathogenic *E. coli* strains, which is passed on to the lambs in the colostrum. This ensures that the lambs are sufficiently protected.

Many *E. coli* strains occur in the intestinal flora of healthy lambs. But if pathogenic *E. coli* strains are ingested, e.g. if environmental conditions are poor and supplies of colostrum are inadequate these types of *E. coli* multiply in the gut. The lining of the gut becomes damaged, leading to diarrhoea.

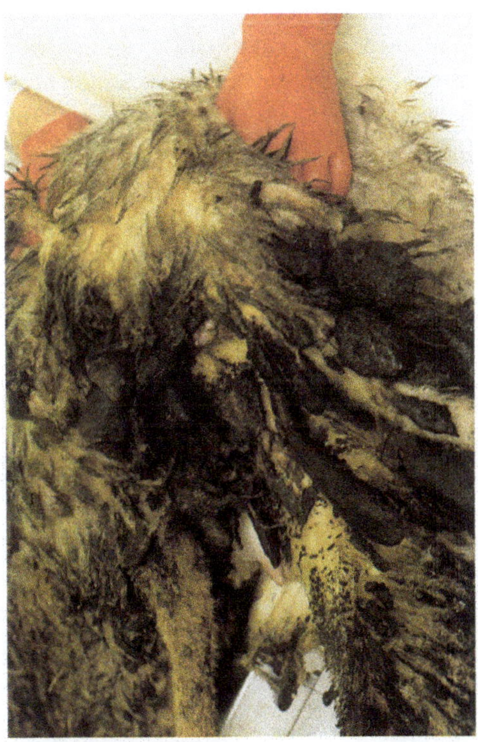

A heavily soiled, clumped fleece following a long episode of scouring

Symptoms: In the first two to three days after birth, lambs become lethargic and often show increased salivation (hence 'watery mouth'). The belly is tucked up and the animal starts to produce greyish-yellow, watery diarrhoea. Lambs die due to fluid loss and the resulting hyperacidity of the blood. The disease lasts only a few days.

Treatment: Treating affected lambs is usually unsuccessful because the fluid loss cannot generally be compensated for in newborns and the antibiotic treatment given is often not specific enough. Laboratory investigations can identify the cause of the diarrhoea so that suitable measures can be taken.

Preventive measures: This disease has multiple causes, making prevention difficult. The most important precaution is to provide the lambs with sufficient colostrum (50 ml several times within the first day of life). The lambing pen should be dry, clean and well ventilated. If diarrhoea does occur, the pen's location should be changed to avoid the increased pressure of infection.

E. coli is ubiquitous in the environment and can never be completely eliminated, so it is vital to reduce the pressure of infection immediately around the animals. Cleaning and disinfection of buildings and lambing pens using suitable disinfectants is helpful in this regard. At lambing time, pay special attention to equipment hygiene in order to avoid transferring pathogens from pen to pen within the house.

Clostridia

Main symptoms

- *Tetanus: spasms, 'sawhorse stance'*
- *Pulpy kidney disease: sudden deaths of well-fed lambs, convulsions, 'downer' animals*

General: Clostridia are spore-forming bacteria. The spores are the permanent form of the pathogen and can occur throughout the animals' environment. They enter the body through injuries and wounds. Once inside, they replicate and produce toxins, which cause typical symptoms. Clostridia also occur in the gut of healthy animals. If animals are not fed appropriately for their species, the bacteria multiply and the toxins produced are distributed to every organ via the bloodstream (enterotoxaemia).

As a result, two types of clostridial infection are distinguished:

1. **Wound infections** with subsequent production of toxins, and
2. **Enterotoxaemia diseases** (increased internal production of toxins).

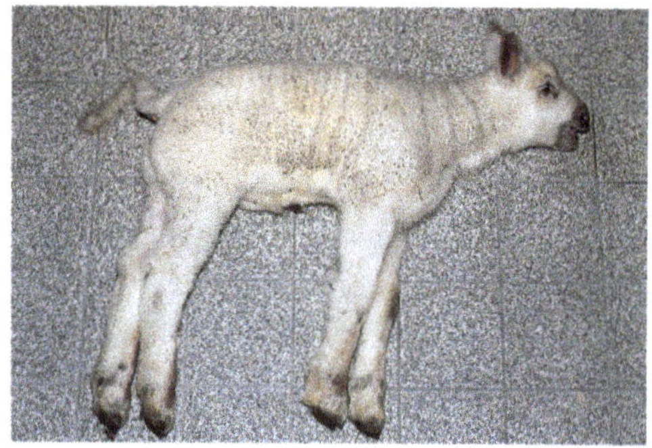

'Sawhorse stance' in a lamb with tetanus

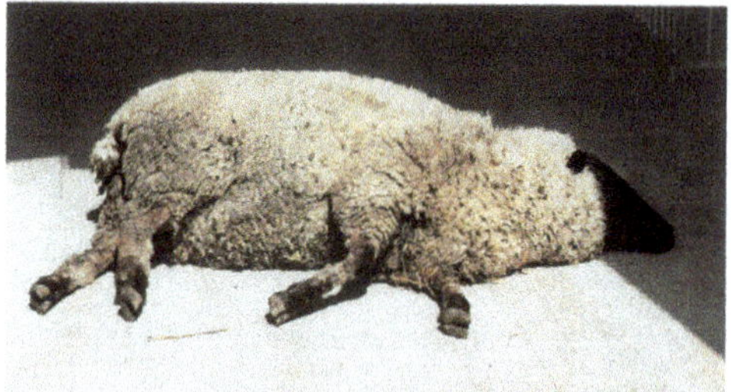

A well-fed 'downer' yearling sheep with paddling leg movements in a case of 'pulpy kidney disease'

Clostridial infections and their symptoms.

Disease	*Symptoms/prevention, treatment*
Wound infections	
Tetanus (*Clostridium tetani*)	– Muscle tremors, stiffness, spasms, 'sawhorse stance'; often after poor navel disinfection in newborns, after castration and tail docking – Vaccination with combined vaccines (tetanus and enterotoxaemia) of ewes and lambs from two to three weeks old – Treatment: pointless
Blackleg (*Clostridium chauvoiei*)	– Bloody, inflamed muscles with gas production – Painful muscle swelling, e.g. birth canal, lower abdomen, pelvic muscles – Confined to a limited region: Northern Germany, Alpine foothills – Treatment: none
Malignant oedema (*Clostridium novyi type A*)	– Often oedema of the vagina and uterus, severe swelling around the wound, fever, discharge often mixed with gas bubbles, foul smelling – Prevention: clean surroundings, wound treatment with antibiotic powders or creams, wound disinfection (iodine); vaccination with combined vaccines – Treatment: prompt administration of high doses of antibiotics
Enterotoxaemia diseases	
Lamb dysentery (*Clostridium perfringens type B*)	– Deaths in one- to three-day-old lambs, short-lasting disease with pain sensitive abdomen, yellowish then brown and bloody diarrhoea – Prevention: 2 x immunisation of dams three weeks before lambing, cleaning and disinfection in lambing house – Treatment: High doses of antibiotics with fluids, usually too late
'Milk colic', enterotoxaemia (*Clostridium perfringens type D*)	– Sudden deaths in well-fed singleton lambs, death in one to 12 hours, is often not recognised immediately – Prevention; see above – Treatment: usually too late
'Pulpy kidney disease' (*Clostridium perfringens type D*)	– Disease with sudden deaths in suckling lambs aged one to two months old and in fattening lambs aged six to 12 months and in adult sheep and goats; affected animals show excess salivation, laboured breathing, convulsions, collapse, 'downer' animals usually associated with ample feeding: high proportion of starch, protein-rich fodder, excessive milk intake, diet low in crude fibre, almost always affects well-nourished animals – Prevention: 2 x immunisation of dams, immunisation of lambs from two to three weeks old, diet high in crude fibre, gradual feed transition – Treatment: almost always pointless

Wound infections	Enterotoxaemia diseases
Tetanus Blackleg	Lamb dysentery Enterotoxaemia ('milk disease') 'Pulpy kidney disease' • Suckling and fattening lambs • One- to two-year-old sheep

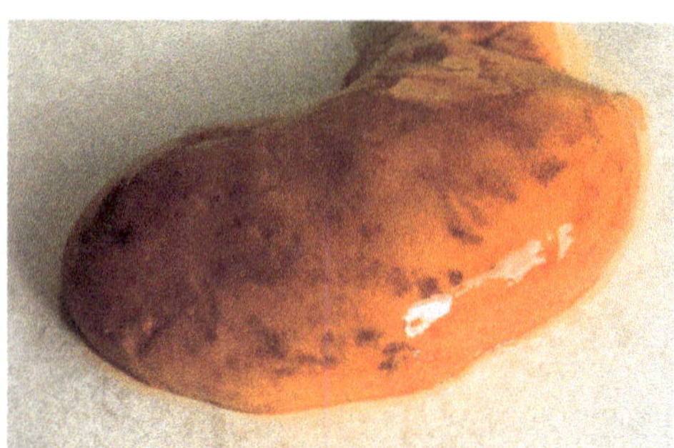

Typical haemorrhages and softening of the kidney = 'pulpy kidney'

Diagnosis: Clostridial infection is diagnosed in a specialist laboratory, where the typical organ lesions can be demonstrated and the pathogen cultured.

Treatment and preventive measures: In acute cases of tetanus, pulpy kidney disease and 'milk colic', treatment is generally unsuccessful.

It is important to take the hygiene measures and to vaccinate appropriately using available vaccines.

Pasteurellosis

Main symptoms

- → *Fever*
- → *Rapid breathing*
- → *Coughing*
- → *Cloudy nasal discharge*

General: Pasteurellosis is the most common form of pneumonia in sheep, affecting lambs in particular. It is growing in importance and causes significant losses in lamb rearing. Pasteurellosis is a major problem for sheep and goat keepers: besides bacteria (Pasteurellae), other pathogens (viruses, mycoplasmas) and environmental stressors also play a role in outbreaks of the disease. Pasteurellosis is therefore described as a 'multi-factorial disease', meaning that multiple factors are involved in its development.

Pasteurellae can be detected in the upper respiratory tract (nose, throat) of almost every sheep but as a general rule do not cause any symptoms. An outbreak occurs only when animals are exposed to various stress factors: feed transitions, changes of pasture, poor ventilation, adverse weather conditions, high stocking densities and accompanying diseases such as worm infestations. These factors impair the body's natural defences, enabling the Pasteurellae to multiply. The bacteria break through the body's defence barriers and the symptoms of pasteurellosis start to appear.

Symptoms: Newborns and older lambs develop a high fever (up to 42°C), restlessness and rapid breathing. Sudden deaths occur without being preceded by symptoms. Older animals display a harsh cough, watery to cloudy nasal discharge with mucus, and laboured breathing. The body temperature

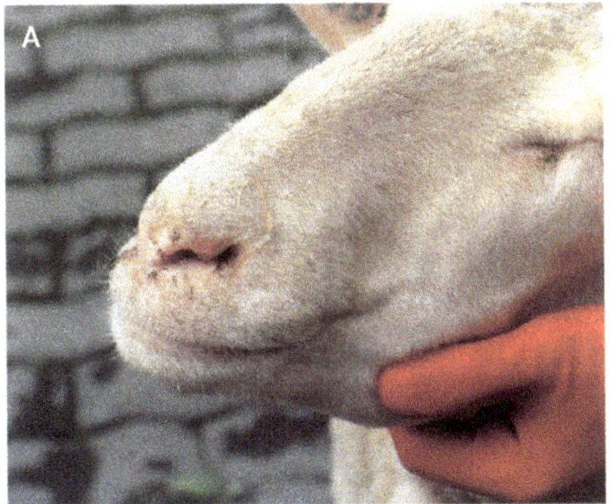

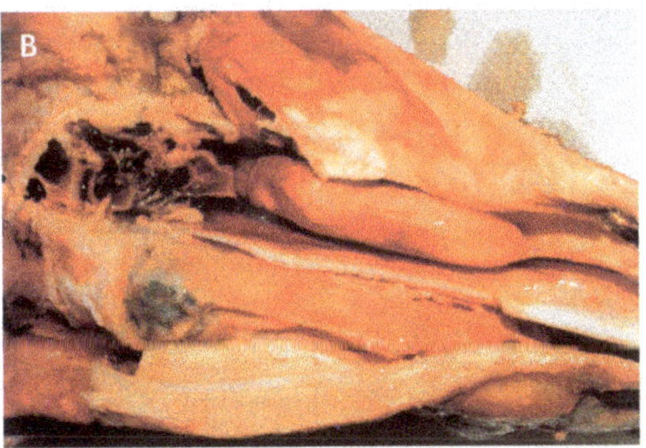

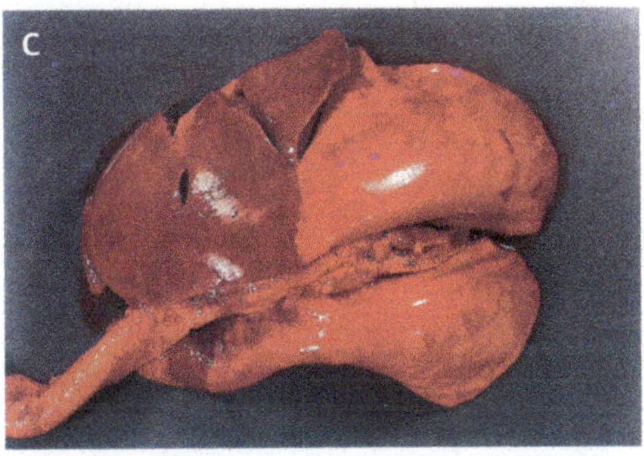

A: dried crusts of cloudy nasal discharge in a sheep with pasteurellosis. B: Pasteurella abscess in the nasal cavity. C: deep red colour and thickened tissue in inflamed areas of lung

rises to 40–41°C. Rustling noises can be heard on listening to the lungs. Younger lambs often die after treatment. In older lambs, the disease takes a chronic form accompanied by emaciation, poor weight gain and a reduced ability to cope with exertion (animals hang back from the flock). At slaughter, the lungs are found to be stuck to the ribs (pleurisy).

Treatment and preventive measures: Stressors should be removed.

All husbandry and feeding changes should be undertaken carefully, with close observation of the animals. In lamb rearing, good ventilation and a low stocking density are important.

Various antibiotics can be used to treat the acute form of the disease. To this end, antibiotic resistance testing is recommended after the bacteria involved have been isolated in the laboratory. Bacteria can be isolated from nasal swabs, pulmonary lesions from slaughtered sheep or the organs of dead animals following post mortem. Once again, it is important to eliminate poor husbandry and environmental conditions.

The **vaccine** currently available has been used with varying degrees of success. It is important to administer the vaccine in accordance with the manufacturer's instructions. Vaccination of dams and regular boosters for lambs are crucial. It is also vital to improve the husbandry conditions. Vaccinating without improving the environmental conditions at the same time is unlikely to succeed.

Brucellosis

Main symptoms

- → *Abortions*
- → *Sickly lambs*

General: Brucellosis, a chronic animal disease caused by *Brucella melitensis*, is widespread in **sheep** and **goats** in the Mediterranean but is less of an issue in the UK.

In rams, *Brucella ovis* infection causes contagious epididymitis. This disease is confined to rams and is not notifiable.

Brucella melitensis infection can be transmitted to humans, cattle, dogs and pigs. It is a zoonosis (**notifiable**!).

Agent	Primary host	Secondary host
Brucella melitensis	Sheep, goat	Human
Brucella ovis	Sheep	

Infection: Typical infection routes include ingestion of the agent via infected afterbirths, water or feed, and transmission during mating. The agent is shed in massive quantities during premature births but can also be shed in milk, urine, dung and nasal discharge.

The disease is introduced to a flock by buying in animals. *Brucella ovis* infection in rams (epididymitis) is passed from ram to ram by direct contact; contaminated dams can infect rams during mating.

Symptoms: A higher abortion rate and births of weak lambs are the most obvious symptoms. However, mastitis, arthritis and inflammation of the testicles and/or epididymes are also observed.

Diagnosis: The symptoms are not particularly specific and need to be confirmed by laboratory examination of stillbirths and premature foetuses, and by means of blood tests.

Epididymitis *(B. ovis)* can be identified by examination and should be confirmed by laboratory tests.

Control: *B. melitensis* infection of sheep and goats is a notifiable disease, so control is carried out by the national veterinary authorities. When buying in animals, it is therefore advisable to have a blood test done.

The introduction of *B. ovis* by breeding rams can be avoided by examining the animals.

The disease in humans

(Brucella melitensis)

Humans can become infected by two routes:

1. Contact with infectious material (stillborn lambs, afterbirths, urine and faeces); the agent enters the body through the skin and mucous membranes.
2. Consumption of infected milk and dairy products.

The symptoms range from general disorders such as fever and sweating, to swollen livers and spleens, and cardiovascular disorders. Chronic forms accompanied by arthritis can also occur. Treatment is not always successful.

People at risk of infection include sheep keepers and veterinarians.

Tuberculosis

Main symptoms

- → *Emaciation*
- → *Caseation of internal organs at slaughter*

General: Tuberculosis is a chronic disease of sheep and goats caused by *Mycobacterium bovis, M. avium* and *M. tuberculosis.*

Sheep and goats generally contract the disease from infected cattle. Wildlife reservoirs such as the badger are mainly responsible for spreading infection.

Symptoms: Because the disease is chronic in nature, the typical lesions in the internal organs (caseous, fatty lumps) are not observed until slaughter. Before then, animals become emaciated despite having a good appetite and show increasing physical deterioration. Sometimes coughing can be heard.

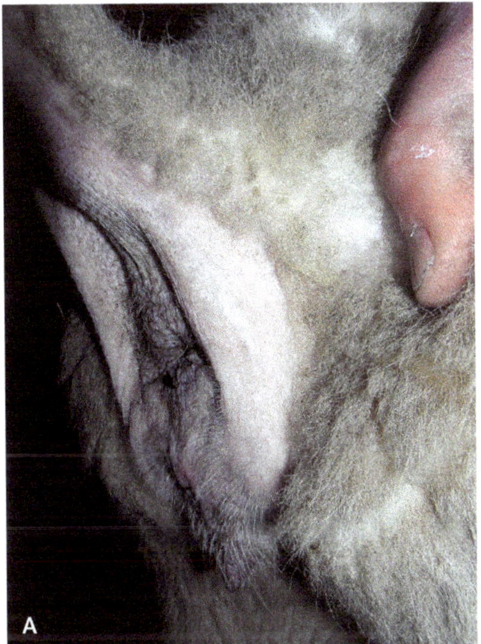

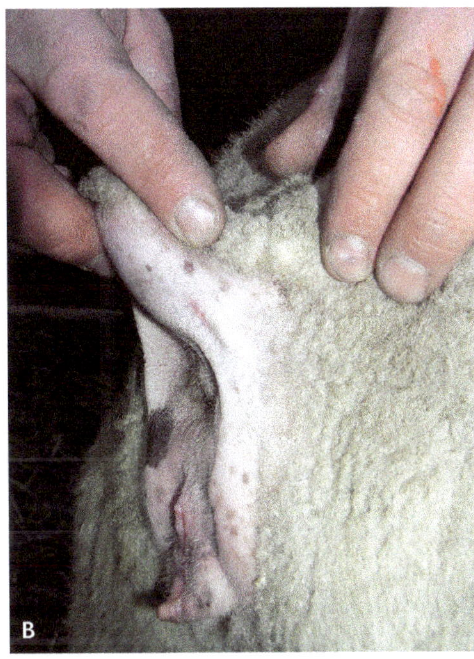

Tuberculin testing: Intradermal test in the anal fold of a sheep. A: negative result. B: a small swelling can be seen soon after the injection

Treatment: Uneconomic.

Tuberculin testing: In some dairy sheep and goat units, animals are tuberculin tested by the veterinary authorities to guarantee their tuberculosis-free status. Tuberculin is injected into the skin of the anal fold beneath the tail. The results are assessed after four days: an increase in skin thickness over 4 mm = positive.

11

Other pathogens

Mycoplasmas

Main symptoms

- *Pneumonia*
- *Arthritis*
- *Mastitis*

General: Mycoplasmas are a group of pathogens that can cause a range of diseases, usually in combination with other agents. They are often involved in pneumonia (chronic pasteurellosis), arthritis and inflammation of the eyelids. Sheep and goats in the Mediterranean are also affected by a disease called **contagious agalactia**, caused by the agent *Mycoplasma agalactiae*.

Symptoms: *Mycoplasma agalactiae* infection in sheep and goats causes inflammation of the udder (mastitis) leading to a lack of milk (agalactia). The infection generally enters the udder via the teat canal. Young animals then contract it from the milk. Infections of the joints and eyes can also occur but these are caused by different mycoplasmas. Inflammation of the cornea and conjunctiva (**keratoconjunctivitis**) can sometimes involve rare species of mycoplasma. **Goats** are more susceptible than sheep.

Diagnosis: These pathogens can only be cultured on artificial nutrient media containing serum, which makes mycoplasma infection difficult to diagnose. Pathogen typing is conducted only in a few specialised laboratories.

Treatment and preventive measures: To avoid introducing contagious agalactia, animals imported from Mediterranean countries must be tested (antibody detection). Those testing positive should be slaughtered. Animals infected with different mycoplasma species can be treated with specific antibiotics.

Note: Not all antibiotics are effective against mycoplasmas!

Q fever

Main symptoms

- *Premature births, isolated or in clusters*
- *Rarely, abortion*

General: Q fever is an infectious disease caused by the **rickettsial organism** *Coxiella burnetii.* In sheep and goats it is usually asymptomatic. The name 'Q fever' comes from the word 'query', reflecting the fact that the agent remained unidentified for a long time.

The infection is especially significant in sheep, as rickettsial agents can be transmitted from sheep to humans.

Symptoms: When pregnant ewes first become infected, the pathogens enter the udder, uterus and amniotic membranes. Births are usually normal; abortions are rare. However, large quantities of the pathogen are excreted during lambing, so other sheep in the flock can become infected in this way. Pathogens can also be detected in the milk of infected animals. Humans are unlikely to contract the infection from milk.

Other symptoms such as lethargy, pneumonia and fever tend to be unclear and are atypical.

Diagnosis: It is important to investigate all premature births, whether isolated or in clusters.

It is also possible to test blood samples. However, acute infections cannot always be detected in this way.

A diagnosis of Q fever in sheep and goats can be made indirectly by means of antibody detection. For this purpose, blood or milk samples are collected from animals in the suspect flock and tested in the laboratory. Special investigation methods (e.g. ELISA) are used to detect the antibodies. Tests like these are especially important for keepers of dairy sheep and goats, as they need to know their animals' Q fever status in order to avoid passing on infection to humans via untreated milk. Milk from infected animals should be pasteurised, and sick or suspect animals should be slaughtered with special precautions and their organs destroyed.

Coxiella is part of the genus Rickettsia, which also includes the agents responsible for spotted fever. These agents cannot be cultured on artificial nutrient media. Under the microscope, however, they can be demonstrated in suitable sample material (afterbirth) using special staining methods.

Treatment: The infection can be controlled with suitable antibiotics but this does not stop the shedding of the pathogen. Nor does it usually prevent abortions.

In cases of Q fever abortion, the flock's location should not be changed. This prevents any further spread of infection and allows protective immunity to develop. Infected non-pregnant sheep do not pose a risk to other animals or humans but can shed the pathogen again the next time they

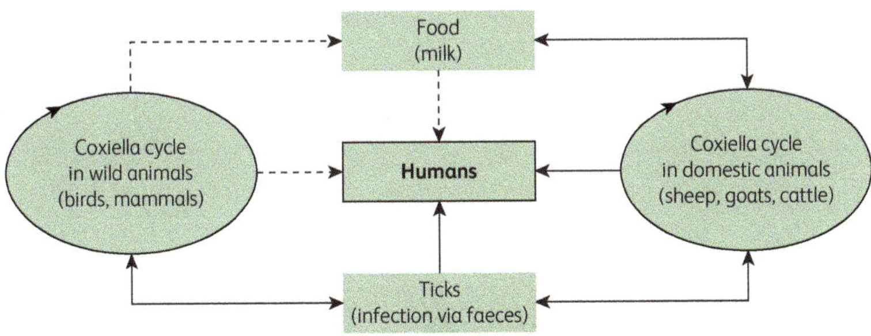

Developmental cycles of Coxiella in wild and domestic animals, and routes of transmission to humans

lamb, helping to spread the infection. Dust from buildings in which infected sheep have lambed, and dried tick faeces in the animals' fleeces, contain huge quantities of infectious material.

Note: Q fever is a **reportable** disease if you are selling milk for consumption.

Infection and symptoms in humans

Humans generally become infected by breathing in dust or airborne droplets containing the pathogen. Substantial quantities of pathogen are needed for the infection to take hold. On the other hand, humans are unlikely to contract the disease by drinking untreated milk from infected sheep or goats. Pasteurising the milk kills enough of the bacteria. The main groups at risk are shepherds, farmers, vets and butchers. In humans, the symptoms appear two to three weeks after infection and include fever (occasionally over 40°C), headaches, chills and atypical pneumonia with a dry cough. However, Q fever infection in humans can also take the form of a mild influenza. A diagnosis of Q fever can be confirmed by blood tests (serology).

12

Protozoan diseases

Generalised infections in sheep and goats caused by single-celled parasites include **toxoplasmosis** *(Toxoplasma gondii)* and **sarcocystosis** (*Sarcocystis* sp.).

Toxoplasmosis

Main symptoms

- → *Abortions*
- → *Stillbirths*
- → *Sickly lambs*

General: Toxoplasmosis is an infection of sheep and goats caused by *Toxoplasma gondii.* Toxoplasmas are single-celled parasites belonging to the Coccidiae. They have sheep and goats as an intermediate host. Kittens are the definitive host.

Sheep and goats become infected by ingesting cat faeces. The main sources of infection are infected pastures, and hay and concentrates contaminated with cat faeces.

Symptoms: Infection in non-pregnant animals rarely causes any symptoms. A first-time infection in the first third of pregnancy leads to resorption of the foetus. Infection at later stages of pregnancy leads – due to infection of the amniotic membranes – to abortions, stillbirths and births of weak lambs.

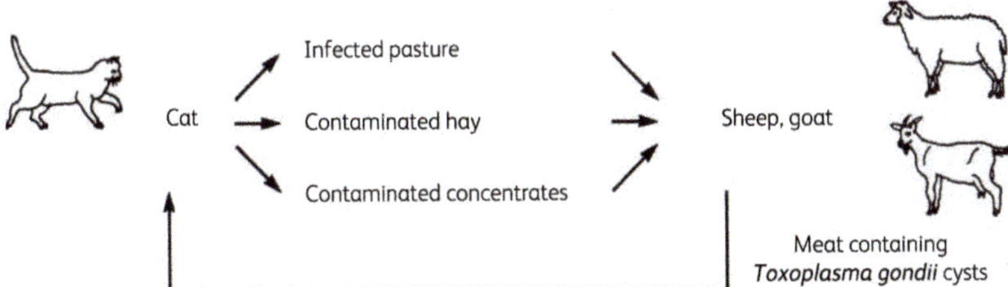

Transmission routes of *Toxoplasma gondii* infection: oocysts excreted in cat faeces are ingested by sheep and goats. Infectious cysts develop in the animals' muscles. The cycle is completed when raw meat containing cysts is fed to cats

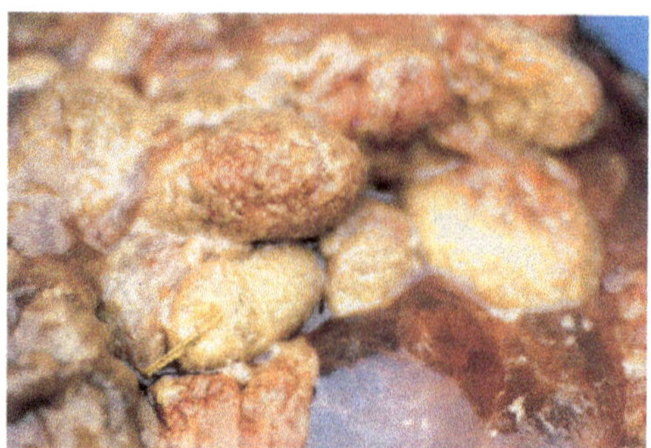

Speckly, slimy afterbirth from a Toxoplasma abortion

Ewes infected before pregnancy usually have robust immune protection, and no pregnancy problems are observed if infection recurs. **Goats**, on the other hand, are susceptible to a second infection and may abort. Dams affected by Toxoplasma abortion appear healthy. Around 12 to 20% of all kid losses are attributable to infection with *Toxoplasma gondii*. In some herds, losses can be as high as 40%.

Preventive measures: To prevent Toxoplasma abortion in sheep and goats, cats should be kept out of pastures, buildings and feed stores (unfortunately, this is usually almost impossible to achieve). Because abortions occur in sheep that become infected during pregnancy without having had previous contact with *Toxoplasma*, newly acquired non-pregnant dams should stay in the flock for a while before being mated. During this time, the sheep can build up natural protection (immunity) by ingesting oocysts in feed contaminated with cat faeces. This immunity then prevents abortion and stillbirths.

Toxoplasmas are fairly resilient organisms, surviving for three weeks in meat at 4°C and for around two years in cat faeces, e.g. on pasture.

Note: Toxoplasmosis is a **zoonosis**, which means that it can be transmitted from animals to humans. There are two routes of infection:

1. oral ingestion of the tiny oocysts in cat faeces (e.g. when cleaning the litter tray),
2. consumption of raw or undercooked meat from animals infected with Toxoplasma. Dogs also become infected but, unlike cats, do not shed any oocysts.

Toxoplasmosis in humans is normally asymptomatic. However, in pregnant women it can cause serious damage to the unborn child. For this reason, pregnant women should abstain from eating raw pork, beef or lamb if they do not have an existing immunity to toxoplasmosis. The doctor can establish this by means of a simple blood test.

It is only a first-time infection during pregnancy that can cause serious harm to the unborn child. Serological blood testing of pregnant women is therefore vital in order to avoid any risk (see above) of infection.

Sarcocystosis

Main symptoms

- → *Few typical symptoms*
- → *Cysts in the muscles and oesophagus on slaughter*

General: Sarcosporidia, which occur in all domestic animals, are also part of the oocyst-forming Coccidiae group. Sheep and goats are intermediate hosts; this means that the cysts form in their muscles. Dogs or cats act as definitive hosts and shed the oocysts in their faeces. Sheep and goats become infected by ingesting the oocysts. The pathogens from dogs pose a greater risk in terms of causing disease.

Symptoms: In sheep and goats, the typical muscle cysts develop in the skeletal musculature, heart muscle and especially the oesophagus. Natural infections in sheep and goats are generally asymptomatic. However, the foci of disease are identifiable on slaughter as cysts in the oesophageal muscles. In many sheep, they can be detected microscopically in the heart muscle. If anaemia, weight loss and abortion are observed in sheep or goats, acute sarcocystosis should be considered as a possible diagnosis.

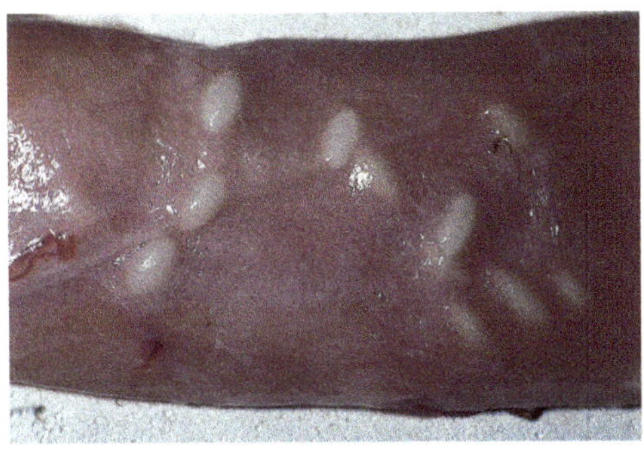

Sarcosporidia cysts on the oesophagus

Preventive measures: To break the cycle of infection, herding dogs should be fed cooked meat only.

13

Diseases of the skin, wool and coat

The skin, with its wool or coat, is the outer covering for the whole body. It protects against injury, dehydration, chemical influences and temperature effects such as heat and cold.

At the same time, it serves as a fat store and has special sensors to record pressure stimuli and fluctuations in temperature. The skin also plays an important role in the body's defence against pathogens. At the body's orifices (mouth, nose, anus, vagina, penis), the skin transitions into mucous membranes. The skin contains hairs, sebaceous glands and sweat glands. Under the top layer (epidermis) is a layer of connective tissue (dermis) with a high density of elastic fibres and collagen fibres. These lend the skin firmness and are the basis for the production of leather.

In sheep, the quality of the wool fibres provides information about the animal's state of health. Pregnancy, nutritional deficiencies, diseases and metabolic disorders lead to poor wool quality by producing a thinner fibre and interrupting wool growth, possibly extending as far as partial or even complete wool loss. Some sheep breeds, such as the Cameroon and Wiltshire Horn, have no fleece. Annual shearing is essential for all wool-bearing breeds on animal health grounds.

External parasites (ectoparasites)

Mites

Main symptoms

- → *Body mange: scratching, rubbing, patchy fleece*
- → *Head mange: skin lesions*
- → *Foot mange: sores and scabs on the forelimb heels, itching*

General: Mites cause various forms of mange in sheep and goats (see below). It is referred to as 'scab' in sheep, ie sheep scab.

Body mange: This disease is normally observed in the winter months (November to February). In sheep, it affects the thickly woolled areas of the neck, back, rump and flanks. Sheep with body mange scratch and rub excessively, lose wool, develop a patchy

Genus of mite	Form of mange	
	Sheep	Goat
Psoroptes	Body mange	Ear mange
Sarcoptes	Head mange	Head mange
Chorioptes	Foot mange	Rare

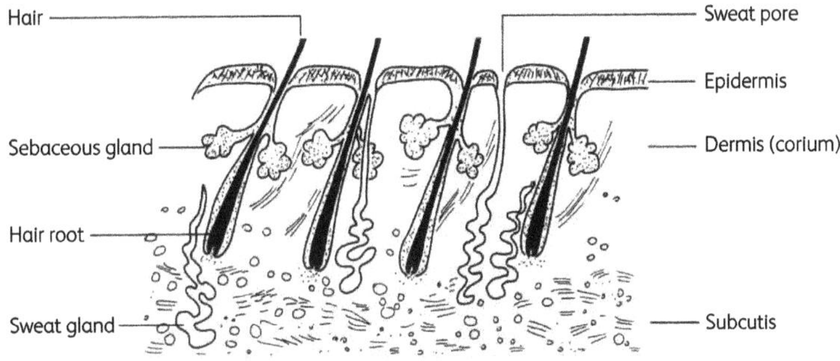

Cross-section of the skin (after Ellenberger and Baum, 1943)

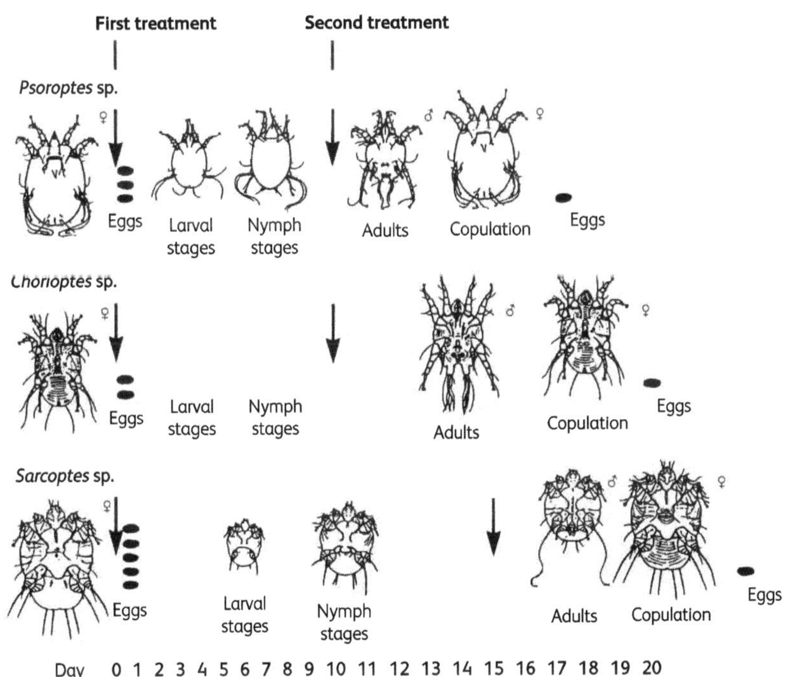

Developmental cycles of different species of mite, with appropriate treatment times. To catch every stage of development requires a second treatment with a suitable control product

appearance, and become emaciated and anaemic.

In goats, the base of the ear is thickened and itchy, and the ear canal becomes blocked with an unpleasant-smelling mass.

Psoroptic mange in sheep is a notifiable disease in UK.

Head mange: *Sarcoptes* mange mites in sheep cause skin lesions on the head and neck. In goats in poor overall condition, the lesions can also extend to the body (ear mange).

Foot mange: The sores and scabs caused by ***Chorioptes*** mites appear on the heels of

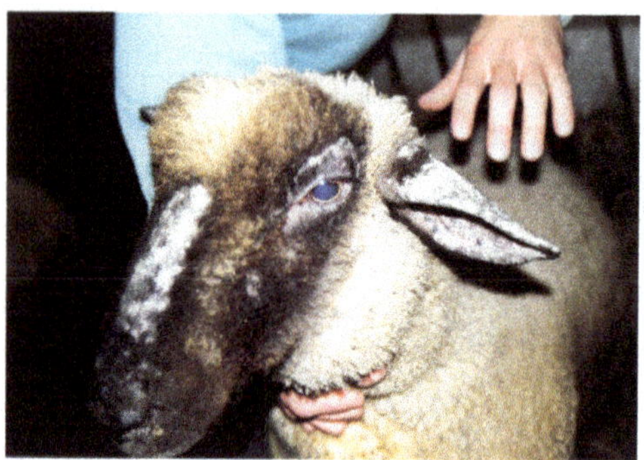

Head mange in a sheep

the forelimbs. Affected animals have a strong urge to scratch. Your veterinary surgeon will diagnose mange by examining a skin scraping for evidence of mites.

Mange control should be tailored to the life cycle of the mite concerned. Treatment takes the form of a dip, spray or injection and should be repeated (in the case of a dip or spray) after one to two weeks. Control should also include the treatment of fences, posts, buildings and pens.

Biting lice

Main symptoms

- *Itching*
- *Wool loss*
- *Visible in fleece*

Biting lice are strictly host-specific ectoparasites which feed on flakes of skin. They need sheep or goats for their survival: separated from their hosts, they can survive for only eight days.

In affected animals, biting lice cause severe itching accompanied by rubbing and loss of wool or hair. Extensive bald patches can develop, with the skin becoming inflamed. Biting lice *(Lepikentron ovis)* measure 1.2 to 1.8 mm in length and are visible in the fleece when it is parted. A magnifying glass can be useful.

Sucking lice

These blood-sucking parasites are rare in sheep and goats. They take around three to four weeks to develop on the animal. Lice can be found in the head and neck area.

Sheep ked

Main symptoms

- *Visible in fleece*

These parasites live in the fleece, usually in sheep and more rarely in goats. Their blood-sucking causes a great deal of irritation to the animal. Sheep keds can transfer to other animals and humans on contact. The highest infestation densities occur in winter. The sheep ked population falls dramatically after shearing.

Ticks

Main symptoms

- *Visible in fleece*

Several species of tick can occur in sheep and goats, including *Ixodes ricinus* (**castor bean tick**) and *Haemaphysalis punctata* (**red sheep tick**). For their developmental cycle, ticks generally need three hosts: they usually start with small rodents (mice, hedgehogs, possibly rabbits, hares, birds) and then move on to larger animals. Ticks can transmit infectious

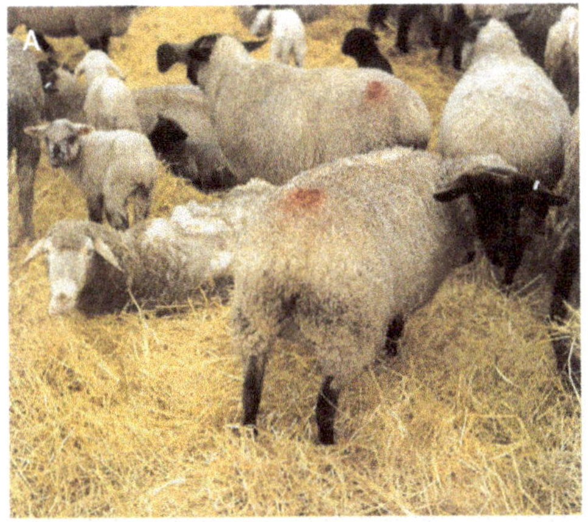

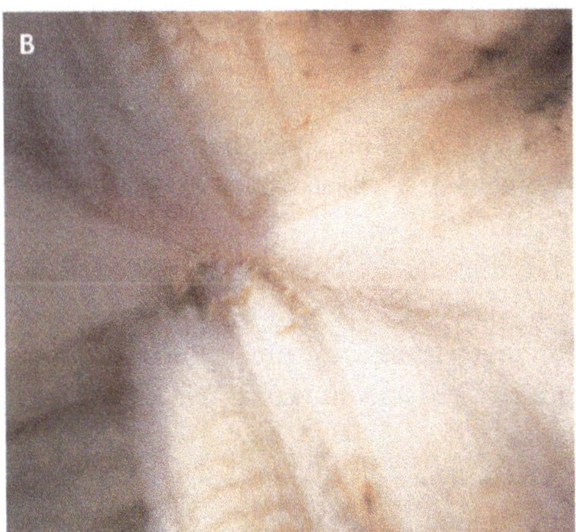

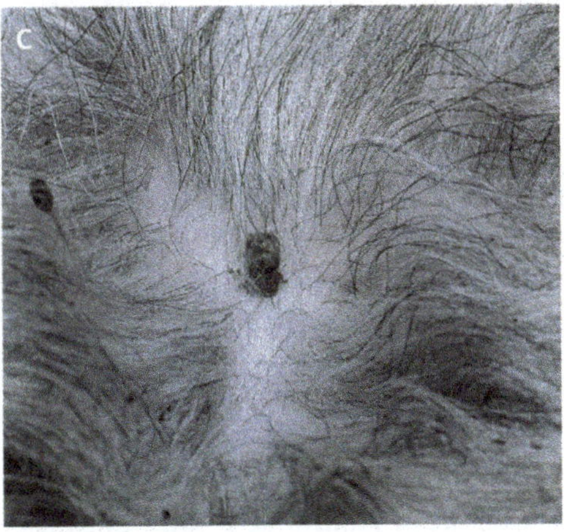

A: In body mange, the fleece appears patchy. B: Scabs and flakes in the parted fleece point to mange. C: Sheep ked in the fleece

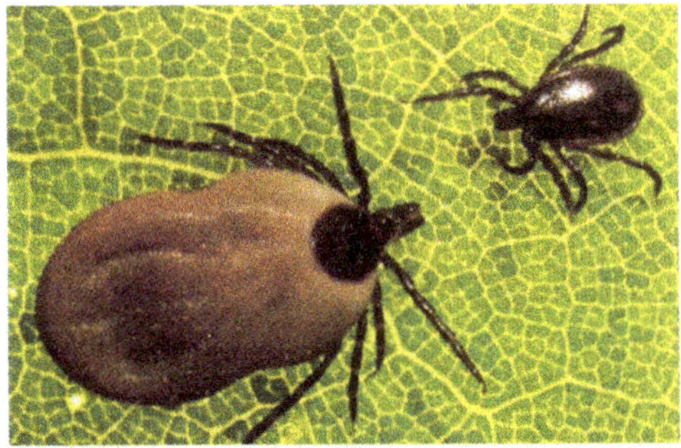

On the left, a female after a blood meal; on the right, a non-engorged tick

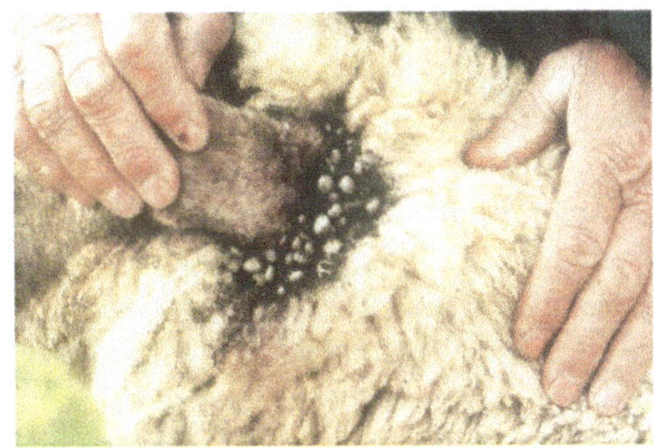

Ticks can transmit Q fever. Large accumulation of ticks around the ear

diseases to humans and animals. In sheep, ticks play an important role as potential carriers of Q fever. In severe tick infestations, animals show restlessness and itching. The ticks are clearly visible in the neck area on parting the fleece.

Fly maggot infestation (fly strike)

Main symptoms

→ *Visible on soiled skin and wool*

Several species of fly lay their eggs on wounds or heavily soiled areas such as the rear ends of animals with diarrhoea. The larvae develop,

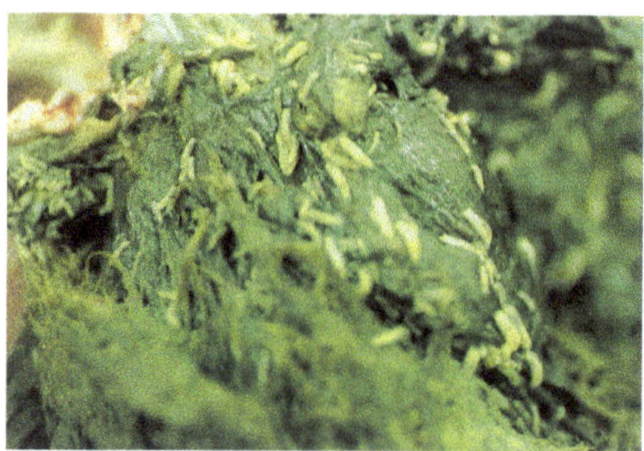

Fly maggots on a badly soiled rear end

penetrate the skin and cause intense skin irritation with a distinctive smell. Thorough cleaning is needed, possibly with shearing of affected areas, as is treatment with insecticides.

Apart from cleaning and insecticides, other measures that can be used to treat an infestation include spraying with chemicals to control external parasites, e.g. chemicals from the avermectins group. However, a new drug specially designed to control fly maggots can only be used preventively as it interferes with the developmental cycle and does not kill the maggots.

Black fly infestation

Under particular climate conditions (warm and damp), swarms of black flies are common in certain river areas. The flies bite sheep and goats on hairless areas of skin (head, testicles, teats). The skin swells and is very painful. Other pasture animals (cows, horses) tend to be affected more often than sheep.

Treatments for ectoparasite infestation

Dip treatment: Bathing or dipping is a good way to control mange mites and other external parasites. It can be done either in a mobile sheep dipper (tank capacity around 3000 l) or in a permanent structure. Mobile dippers can be hired from private operators.

Animals should be well watered and not over-fed before dipping. Dipping of anxious, tired and thirsty animals should be avoided at all costs. Weather conditions should be favourable (dry) because an already wet fleece reduces the effectiveness of the dip.

The best time to dip is around six to eight weeks after shearing. By then the wool will have grown a little, helping the dip to stay in the fleece, but be short enough for good penetration. The animals should stay in the dipper for at least a minute and, for best effect, the dip should be at least at ambient temperature. Both body and head should be submerged; the head may need to be washed separately.

If the flock is badly soiled, dirty areas of skin should be cleaned first to avoid introducing pathogens from the dirt into the dip and possibly transferring them to other animals.

Note: The dip should be mixed thoroughly and topped up with a double-strength concentration after every 100 animals or so, because each fleece soaks up more active ingredient than liquid. When using the preparations listed here, always comply with the precautions and withdrawal periods indicated by the manufacturer.

Spray treatment: With smaller numbers of animals or where dipping is not practicable, sheep and goats can be treated by spraying. Products should be used at double strength (compared with dipping) and ideally sprayed at a pressure of around 5 bar. This method of treatment is not recommended for mange (sheep scab) control as it does not reach all affected areas of skin. Spraying generally gives sufficient control of other external parasites as well.

In this case too, treatment should ideally be carried out between six and eight weeks after shearing and in dry weather. If necessary, it should be repeated.

Washing treatment: Where parasites (e.g. maggots) are confined to isolated areas of the body, another option is to wash these areas only. It is important to start with thorough cleaning, shearing of dirty wool, and the removal of scabs and other deposits. The product should be applied at double strength (compared with dipping) using an applicator such as a sponge. This method only removes parasites from the areas treated. It will not affect parasites at other sites.

Pour-on treatment: On holdings with small numbers of livestock, it is often necessary to treat individual animals. The dip solution is prepared at double strength and, after parting the fleece, is poured along the animal's back from neck to tail head using a watering can. This ensures that the product is distributed over both sides of the body and runs down through the fleece towards the belly. This method is not suitable for mange control but has a satisfactory effect against other parasites, especially if repeated after a couple of weeks.

Powder treatment: This method of treatment is only suitable for individual animals but has the advantage that it can be carried out in winter. In this method, the sheep or goat is treated using a commercial powder insecticide, with the powder being distributed thoroughly over wool and coat. Of course, the product does not reach external parasites or mange mites that are deep down in the fleece. It can only reduce a parasite infestation, not eliminate it completely.

For the treatment of external parasites in sheep, dipping is superior to all of the other methods outlined above. In special cases, depending on local circumstances and the type of holding, one of the other methods described can be used.

Injection treatment: With the introduction of macrocyclic lactones eg avermectins, for the treatment of gastrointestinal worms, there are now drugs on the market that can be used to treat mange by injection. This holds out the possibility of carrying out effective mange treatment in the winter months. However, these drugs' effectiveness is limited in the first instance to the treatment of mites. Other external parasites cannot be controlled sufficiently on account of their life cycles and feeding habits.

It is important to take note of and comply with the directions, dosages and withdrawal periods indicated by the manufacturer.

Further information on the use of the various methods and options for treating ectoparasite infestations can be obtained from your local sheep health service.

Fungal skin infections, 'rain scald' and other infections

Fungal skin infections

Main symptoms

- *Flaky circles on exposed areas of skin*

General: Fungal skin infections are also known as dermatomycoses or ringworm. They are rare in sheep and goats, and often affect only a few animals. Agents include *Trichophyton* sp. and *Microsporum* sp.

Infection: Infection is spread by animal-to-animal contact. The fungal agent can also be assumed to be present in the wool or coat of sheep and goats that are not showing any specific symptoms. Poor hygiene, poor ventilation, lack of vitamin A and other trace elements, and incorrect feeding, all help to spread fungal diseases within the flock. Goats are more susceptible than sheep, and tend to suffer more acutely. The skin lesions are also slower to heal in goats. Sometimes the infection can only be seen in the kids.

Symptoms: Hairless circles of skin are seen on areas not covered by wool (head, ears, limbs). There may also be blood due to increased rubbing activity.

Diagnosis: Fungal culture in the laboratory of skin samples from affected areas.

Treatment: Generally, treatment is by topical application of an antimycotic product. This will need to be repeated. Often, it is sufficient to eliminate deficiencies, lack of vitamins or trace elements, or poor husbandry conditions. Goats can be sensitive to some anti-fungal medications, so treatment for goats should be administered carefully.

Note: The skin fungus *Trichophyton* sp. can also infect humans, so take special care when handling animals with a suspected infection.

'Rain scald'

Main symptoms

- → *Crusting and sloughing in the back and loin region*

General: 'Rain scald' or 'lumpy wool' is a skin disease caused by **bacteria** *(Dermatophilus congolensis)*. It is accompanied by eczema.

Symptoms: After long periods of wet weather and heavy rainfall, some sheep display crusting and sloughing of the fleece, especially in the back and loin region. The thick scabs cause the fleece to become matted. Underneath the scabs, the skin is red and appears inflamed. In many cases, the bacteria responsible have been present on the sheep

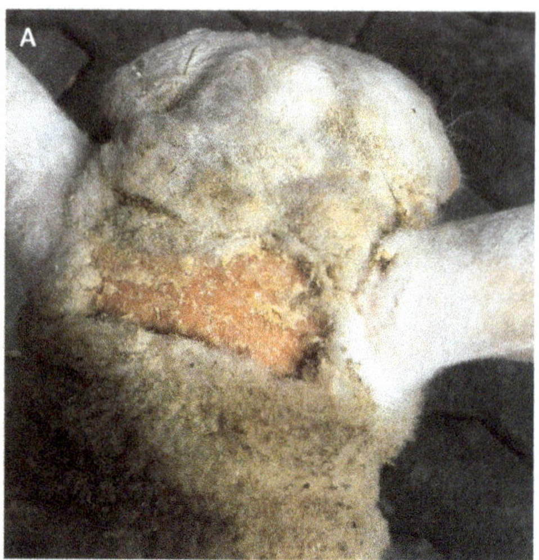

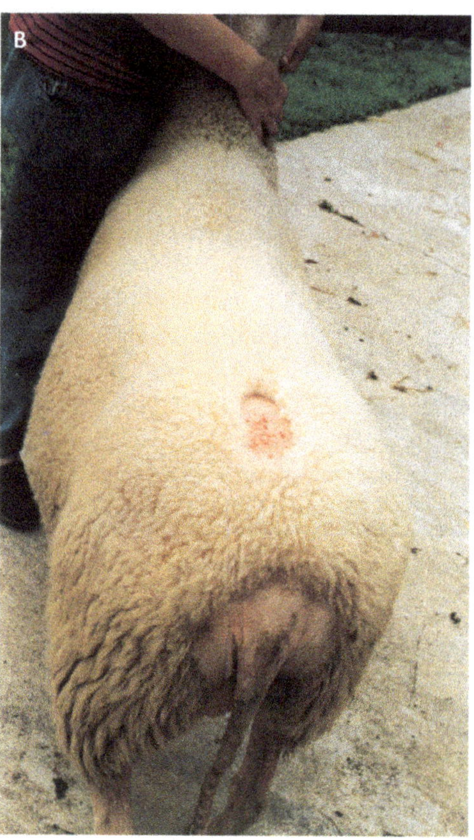

A: Scabbed, reddened area of bare skin on the head; a fungal infection was later diagnosed.
B: 'Rain scald' with scabs and sloughed fleece

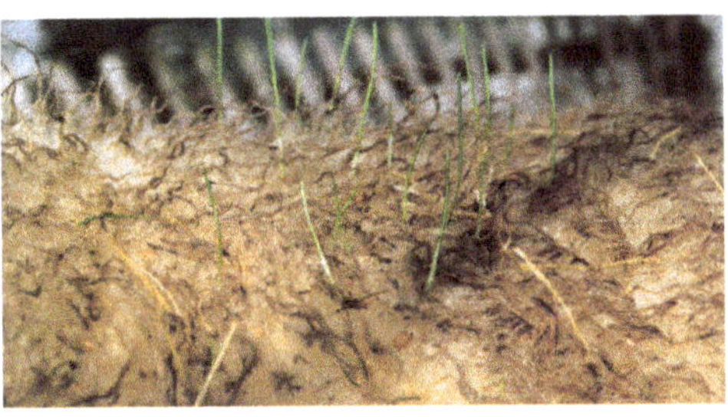

Cereal shoots in a dirty fleece

for some time but only trigger the disease when the skin has been damaged by a long spell of wet weather. Although rare in the UK, in goats the disease affects young animals and animals with longer coats. It usually affects the head and ears, or the inguinal (groin) area. The hairs are encrusted and sloughing of the reddened skin can be seen. Extensive scab formation is a later symptom.

Diagnosis: A 'sticky tape' sample is taken from the affected areas and the pathogen is detected in the laboratory under a microscope.

Treatment and preventive measures: A mild disinfectant solution applied topically to affected areas and, in more serious cases, injections of penicillin/streptomycin have proved invaluable as methods of treatment. Sheep that develop 'rain scald' repeatedly should be removed from the flock as they act as a source of infection for other animals.

Other skin infections

General: Certain types of 'pus-causing' bacteria (Staphylococci) can cause skin infections (pyoderma) which usually occur in areas not covered by wool. These bacteria can also be detected following a viral infection (Orf), in conjunction with fungal infections, or in cases of 'rain scald'.

Treatment: Antibiotic creams, powders or suspensions are applied topically to affected areas of skin. Treatment must be repeated until the infection has cleared up.

Wool eating

General: Although very rare in the UK, eating other animals' wool can be a 'vice' or bad habit in lambs, and usually a sign of deficiency in adult sheep.

Symptoms: Intensively reared lambs nibble other animals and swallow their wool. By clumping together with other foods in the rumen and abomasum, the wool can form hairballs, which then lead to digestive disorders. There are no signs of skin infections or itching in the animals affected. Due to the resulting digestive disorders, lambs lose a lot of weight, become anaemic and suckle less. Their abdomens are often distended. In lambs, this vice usually starts at around two to four weeks old when they eat the wool around their mother's udder and tail. In adult sheep, it tends to be the soiled wool around the tail and hindquarters that is eaten first.

Diagnosis: To identify a potential deficiency in adult sheep, specific blood tests should be carried out. Wool-eating lambs should be removed from the flock to stop other lambs copying this vice.

14

Diseases of the eyes, ears and nervous system

The **eye** receives incoming light and processes it in a light-sensitive layer of sensory cells called the retina. Sheep and goats are able to see colours and distinguish between light and dark.

The **ear**, consisting of the outer, middle and inner ear, receives sound waves, which are perceived as a tone or noise. The outer ear (pinna) acts like a funnel, collecting the sound waves and directing them via the eardrum and middle ear (with its auditory bones) to nerve cells in the inner ear.

The **central nervous system (CNS)**, which consists of the brain, spinal cord and nerves, is one of the most important and most complex organs in the body. It monitors and regulates the functions of the entire organism. Its tasks include:

- Monitoring the internal organs (processes and interrelationships),
- Processing reports from the environment and the internal organs,
- Directing appropriate behaviour.

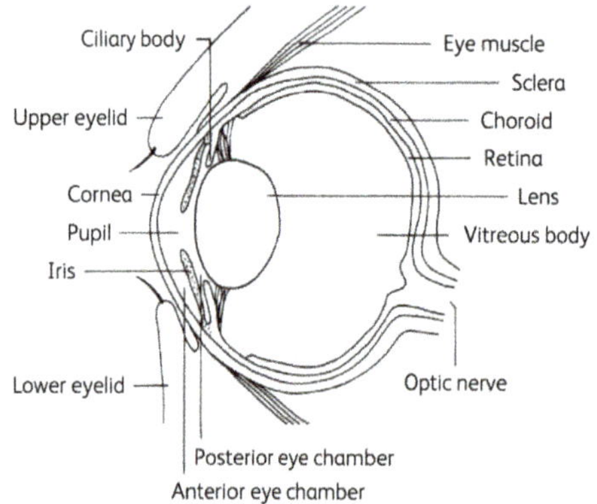

Cross-section of an eyeball

Contagious ophthalmia (pink eye)

Main symptoms

- *Corneal opacity*
- *Reddening of eyelids*

General: Contagious inflammation of the cornea and conjunctiva in sheep and goats is caused by Chlamydia. Other agents such as bacteria and mycoplasmas may also be involved.

The disease is introduced into a flock by asymptomatic carriers or by contact with affected animals from other flocks. Within a flock, Chlamydia is spread by direct contact

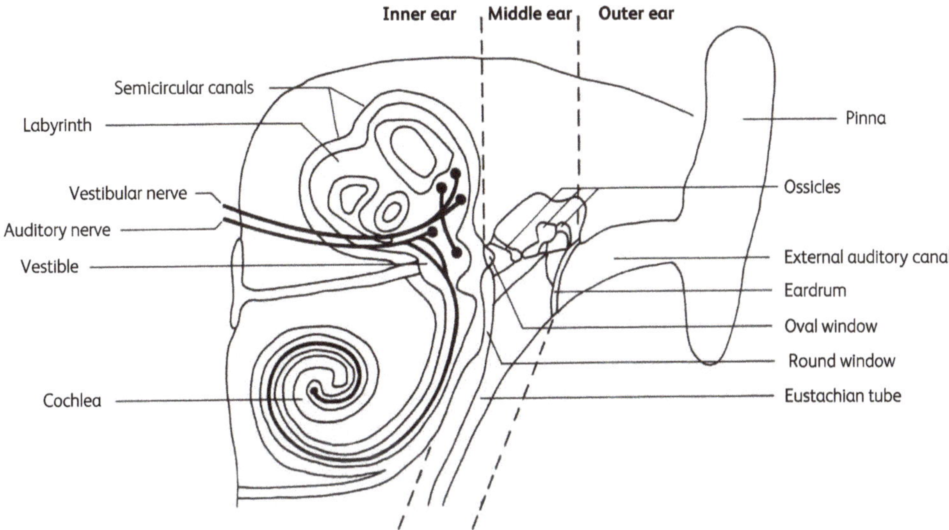

Diagram of the ear

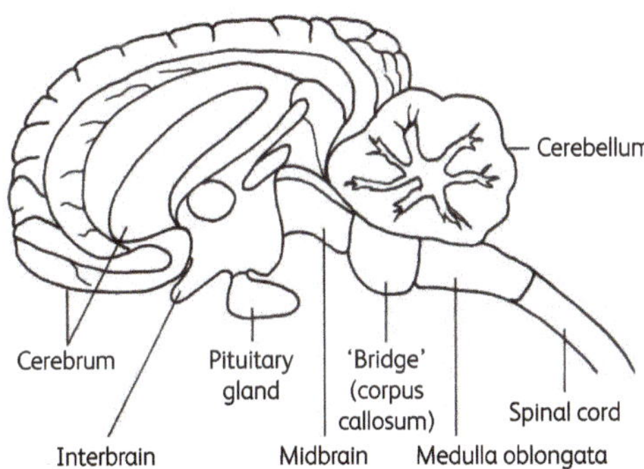

Diagram of the brain (medial section) (according to Nickel, Schummer, Seiferle, 2003)

or by flies out at pasture or in the animals' buildings.

Symptoms: Around a week after infection, animals develop an eye discharge and reddening of the eyelids. The cornea becomes cloudy with white spots.

Diagnosis: The agent can be detected in the laboratory by examining a corneal smear under a microscope. As a rule, especially if a sticky eye discharge is present, bacteriological tests are also recommended.

Treatment: Multiple applications of antibiotic ointment or eye drops (containing tetracyclines). Fly control in buildings is recommended to prevent the disease from spreading. The stocking density should be reduced. Affected animals are a source of infection and should be isolated from the rest of the flock.

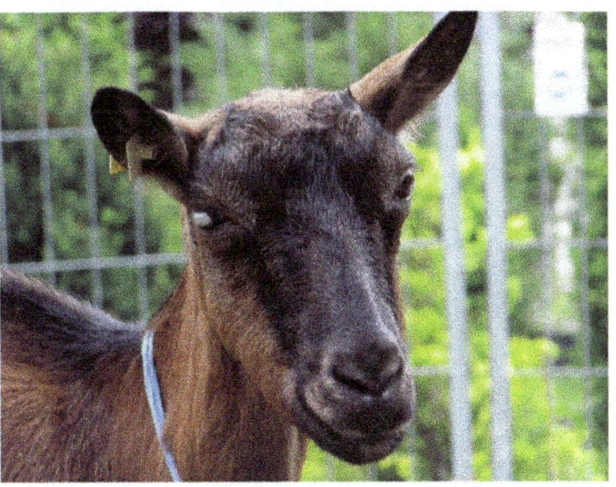

Corneal opacity with white spots following Chlamydia infection

Eye injuries

General: Eye injuries can be caused by grains of cereal, a poke from a horn, or sharp objects such as wood splinters. Pregnancy toxaemia and some types of poisoning can also result in impaired vision.

Treatment: Superficial injuries to the cornea can be cleaned by washing with a gentle solution. An antibiotic ointment protects against more serious infection.

In the event of a deep injury to the cornea, the animal must be brought indoors and the affected eye treated with an antibiotic ointment containing vitamin A. In such a case, always call a vet. It is not correct to use an ointment containing cortisone. Failure to spot an injury promptly or treat it appropriately can result in blindness or loss of the eye.

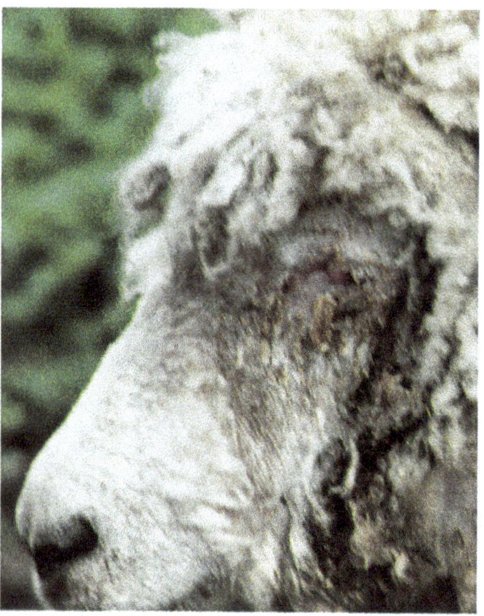

Dog bite injury leading to infection, discharge and loss of the eye

Ear infections

Main symptoms

- *Head tilt*
- *Hypersensitivity to pain*

General: An infection of the ear can affect the outer, middle and/or inner ear. Infections are caused by several kinds of bacteria. Infection can spread from the outside to the inside if not spotted promptly and treated appropriately.

Infections of the outer ear are normally seen after dipping.

Symptoms: If an infection spreads to the middle ear, the animal will droop, tilt or shake its head. The ears become hypersensitive to pressure. If the infection continues to the inner ear (where the organs of balance are located), the animal can develop problems with its balance and movement.

Treatment and preventive measures: Infections of the outer ear are treated by administering antibiotic solutions into the ear canal. A repeat treatment is recommended.

In a middle ear infection, the vet will also have to inject antibiotics. If the animal is already showing problems with its balance and movement, the infection has spread to the inner ear and treatment will be unsuccessful.

Note: Dipping is often at the root of ear infections in sheep, so always use a clean dip and hold the animals' ears closed when submerging their heads, to make sure that no liquid enters the ear canal.

Circling disease (*Coenurosis, 'Gid'*)

Main symptoms

- → *Circling behaviour*
- → *Head tilt*

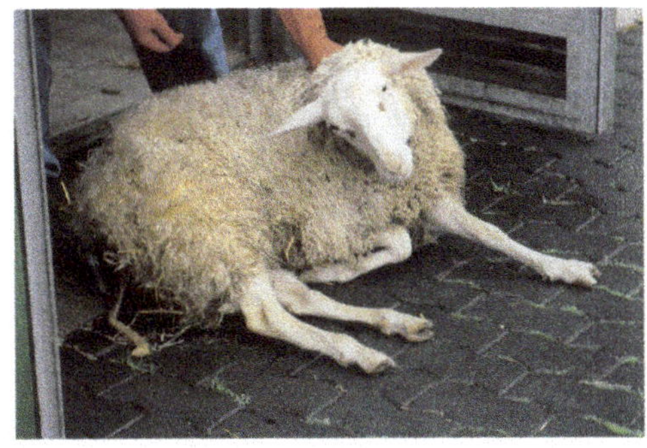
Lowered, tilted head position in circling disease

General: The larvae (developmental stages) of the **dog tapeworm** *(Taenia multiceps)* can migrate to the brain and spinal cord in sheep and goats, causing various movement disorders.

Dogs excrete tapeworm eggs and segments ('proglottids') in their faeces. Sheep and goats then swallow these while grazing. The tapeworm larvae which hatch from the eggs are distributed within the body via the bloodstream and develop into cysts in the brain and, more rarely, in the spinal cord. As the cysts grow, they put pressure on parts of the nervous tissue.

Symptoms: Symptoms include disorientation, agitation, circling movements and head tilting.

Diagnosis: A definite diagnosis can be obtained only by conducting a post mortem on the dead animal.

Treatment: Treatment is generally pointless even though the disease is possible to diagnose in the live animal.

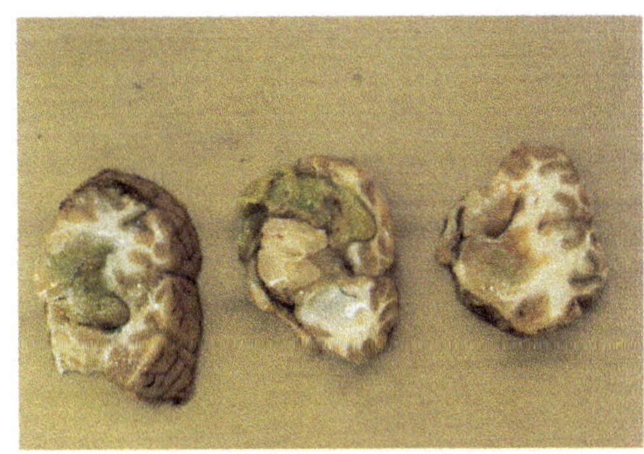
Typical lesions in brain sections from a sheep with circling disease

Preventive measures: The most important measure is regular worming of all dogs (herding dogs, farm dogs, guard dogs) to control tapeworms. Contact with outside dogs should be avoided if possible. New dogs

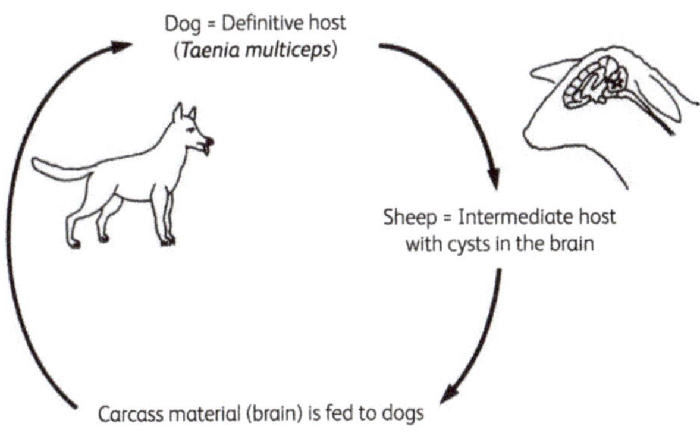

Grazing sheep and goats swallow tapeworm eggs which develop into cysts (= larvae) in the brain, causing the typical symptoms of circling disease. Dogs become infected by eating carcass material. The tapeworm grows inside the dog, which in turn excretes the eggs in its faeces. This closes the cycle. The cycle can be broken by worming your herding dogs and cooking carcass material before feeding it to them

should be wormed before being put to work. Fresh, uncooked sheep carcasses should not be fed to dogs as this continues the tapeworm's life cycle.

The most common tapeworm found in dogs *(Dipylidium caninum)* does not produce cysts in sheep and goats; it uses arthropods (fleas) as an intermediate host.

Below is an overview of **central nervous diseases** of sheep and goats.

Overview of central nervous diseases of sheep and goats (after Dedié and Bostedt, 1996).

Disease	*Agent*	*Symptoms*
Contagious		
Aujeszky's disease (pseudorabies)	Virus	Acute progression, itching, usually contracted from pigs
Rabies	Virus	Excitability, deranged appetite, atypical behaviour, swallowing difficulties
Maedi-visna CAE (caprine arthritis encephalitis)	Virus	Chronic progression, deranged appetite, CAE with swollen joints, maedi with lung disease
Scrapie	Prion protein	Chronic progression, typical 'trotting' gait
Listeriosis	Bacterium	Acute progression, listlessness, usually associated with silage feeding
Non-contagious		
Calcium deficiency		Acute progression, muscle tremors, convulsions while lying on side, usually last third of pregnancy, early lactation
Magnesium deficiency		Acute progression, muscle tremors, convulsions while lying on side, usually after turnout to pasture
Pregnancy toxaemia		Swaying gait, deranged appetite, sternal recumbency, coma, final stages of pregnancy, low blood sugar
Copper deficiency		Usually affects lambs; chronic progression, listlessness, paralysis of hind limbs, later extending to forelimbs

15

Diseases of the bones and joints

Bones come in different shapes: long, hollow bones in the limbs; flat bones in the head, shoulder blade and pelvis. The bones are connected by **joints**.

The **passive musculoskeletal system** (bones, joints and ligaments) and the **active musculoskeletal system** (muscles, tendons and tendon sheaths) together lend stability to the body and enable it to move.

In sheep and goats, the front and hind limbs end in **hooves**.

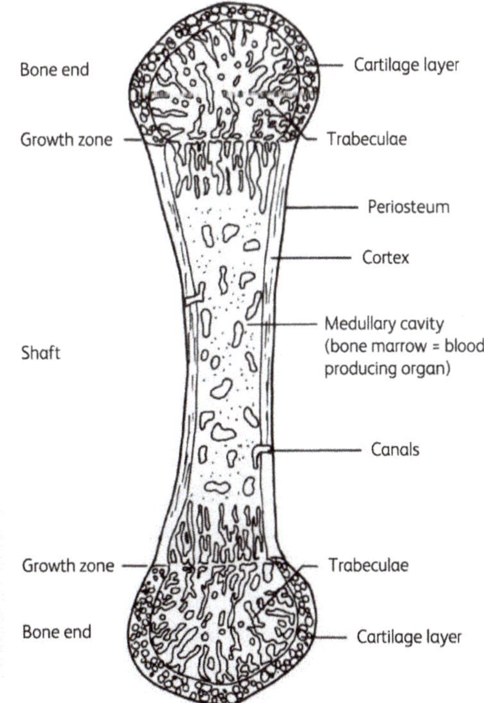

Structure of a hollow bone

Foot rot (infectious pododermatitis)

Main symptoms

- *Lameness*
- *Walking on the knees*
- *Painful swelling between the toes*

General: Foot rot is a transmissible infectious disease of sheep accompanied by inflammation of the hoof laminae and leading to lameness and general poor health. Skin, tendons and bones can also become infected.

Foot rot has a variety of causes, both specific and non-specific. The **specific agents** are two genera of bacteria (*Dichelobacter* spp.

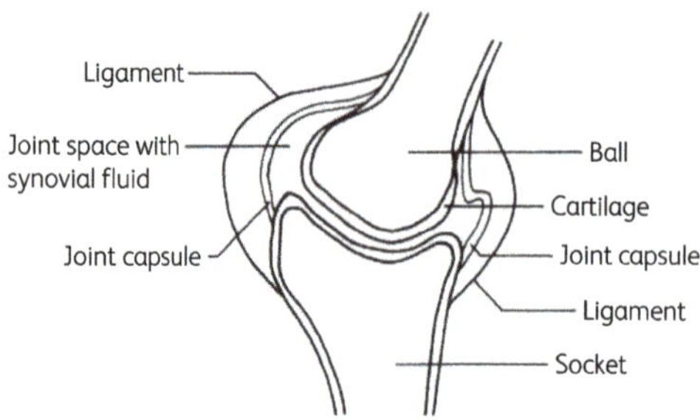

Diagram of a joint in flexed position

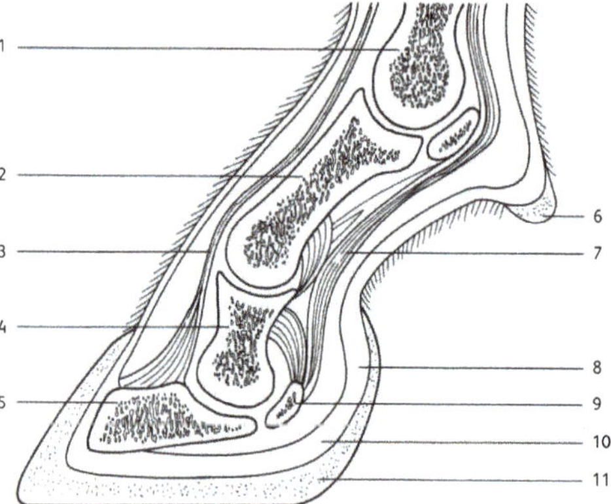

Structure of the sheep's hoof: 1 = Shin bone, 2 = Long pastern bone, 3 = Extensor tendon, 4 = Short pastern bone, 5 = Pedal bone, 6 = Dew claw, 7 = Flexor tendon, 8 = Corium, 9 = Navicular bone, 10 = Sole corium, 11 = Hoof horn

(*nodosus*) and *Fusobacterium* spp.). Infection with both agents leads to inflammation and breakdown of the hooves. *Bacteroides* bacteria remain infectious outside the animal's body for only a few hours but can survive for up to three years in affected hooves. The other agents (*Fusobacterium* spp.) also occur in the soil and are therefore extremely widespread. Because the bacteria survive well in the hoof and are common in the environment, foot rot can persist within a flock for a long time and cause serious financial losses.

A variety of **non-specific factors** can encourage the disease and help bacteria to stick to the hoof. They include high stocking densities, damp bedding, new driving routes, injuries, and poor hoof care.

Symptoms: Around ten days after contact with the pathogen, and in the presence of the non-specific factors mentioned above, the first symptoms appear. They include inflammation of the coronary band with horn separation

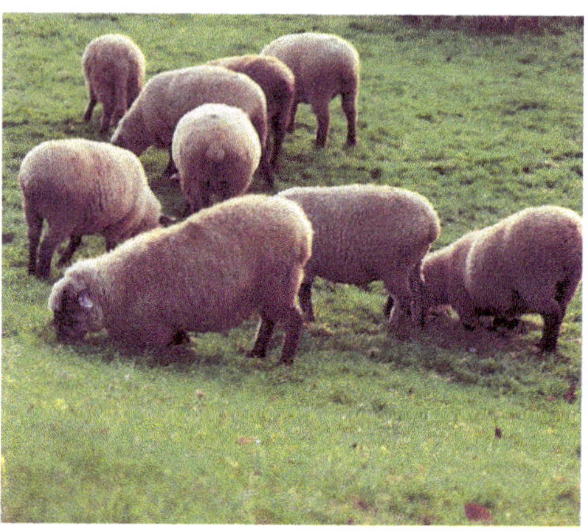

Severe hoof pain causes sheep to walk or graze on their knees

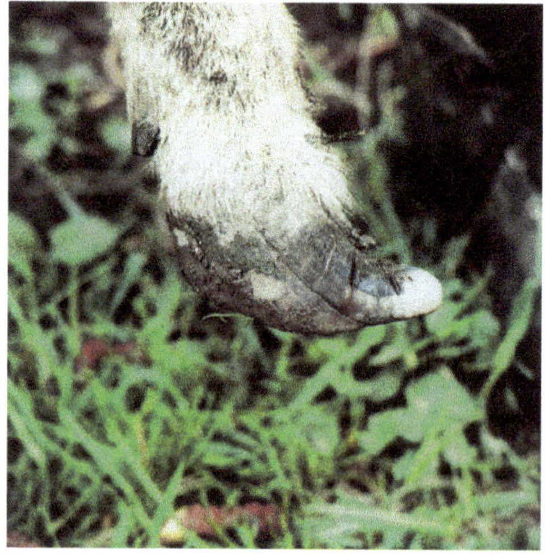

Poor hoof care leads to deformities

and swollen, reddened skin between the toes. As the infection progresses, a painful swelling develops between the toes, around the coronary band and on the sole of the hoof. The sheep go lame on one or more limbs. A foul-smelling greyish white pus builds up in the affected areas. Animals walk or graze on their knees. Their appetite is affected, leading to weight loss and poor wool quality. The animals' immune systems are weakened, making them more susceptible to other diseases.

Treatment: As a first step, all of the sheep in the flock should be examined thoroughly. Local hoof treatments can then be applied, supported by injections.

After trimming the hoof, the antibiotic is applied. This can be in the form of a spray, ointment (mastitis tubes) or powder. However, current UK data indicates that trimming retards healing of foot rot cases, and treatment by injection gives the best response.

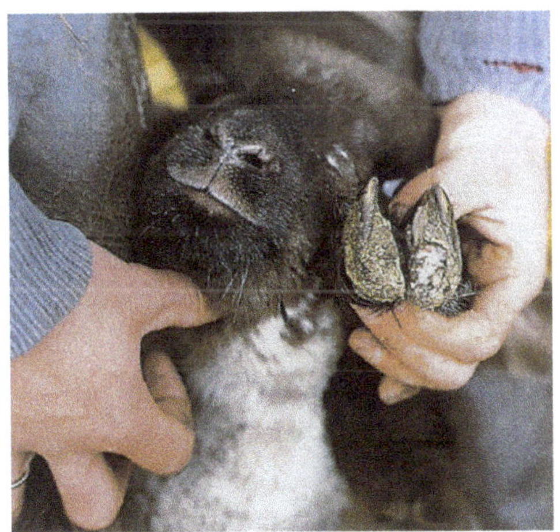

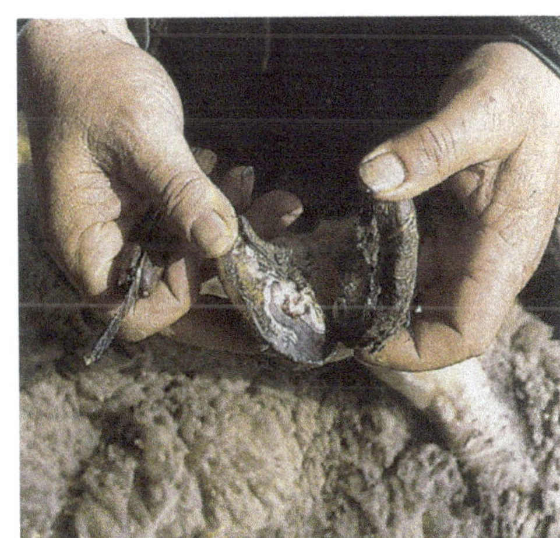

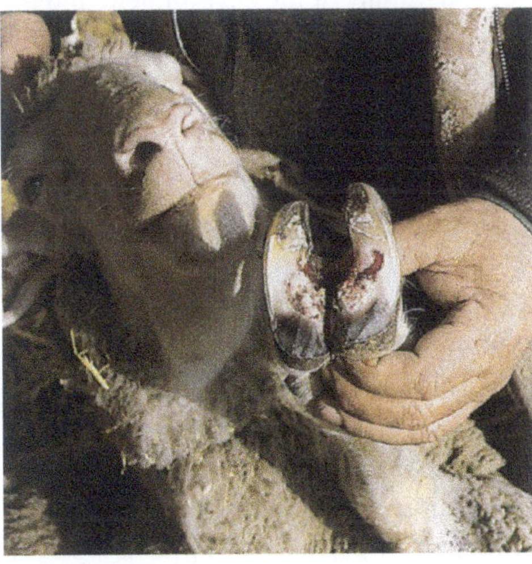

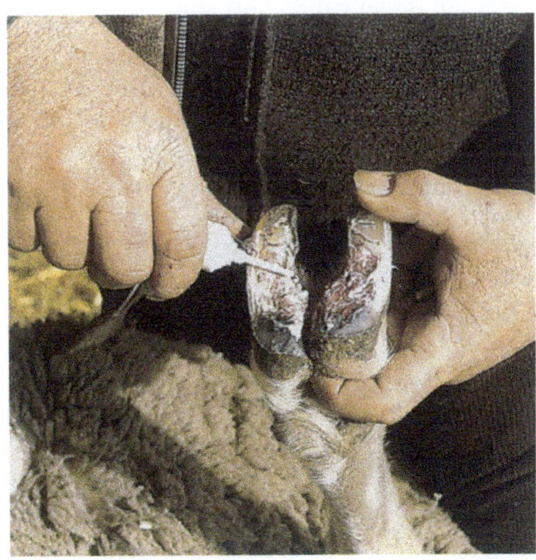

In this sequence of photos, loose horn and dead tissue are removed using a sharp knife, the affected tissue is exposed and the hoof is treated with an antibiotic ointment

Dipping in a 10 to 20% zinc sulphate solution or a special hoof dip has a disinfectant effect. Toxic substances such as copper sulphate or drugs containing arsenic should no longer be used for treatment purposes. In addition to this local treatment, your vet can inject antibiotics to combat the bacteria responsible for foot rot.

If the disease is widespread within the flock, treatment can be expensive and time-consuming. Foot rot can be eradicated only by combining treatment of individual sheep with measures to protect healthy or recovering animals.

Preventive measures: Weekly hoof dipping using a disinfectant and some household detergent has proved effective.

Krevol solution is tolerated well and is another option. The sheep should be left to stand on a hard surface for half an hour afterwards to allow the dip to take effect. The success of treatment depends largely on the sheep keeper and on changes to the husbandry conditions.

Note: Protective vaccination with a foot rot vaccine helps to support treatment but does not replace hoof care and other animal health measures.

If a vaccine is used, all animals in the flock, including rams and weaned lambs (at least four weeks old), must be included in the vaccination programme. The basic immunisation requires two vaccinations separated by an interval of four to six weeks. The manufacturer recommends a booster after six months. This should be given around six weeks before the time of peak risk.

To protect a healthy or recovered flock against (re-)infection, weekly hoof dipping should be practised after contact with affected animals or in periods of heavy rainfall. Newly bought-in animals should be kept in quarantine for at least two weeks. Their hooves should be examined and, if necessary, treated and dipped.

Summary of foot rot control measures

- → *Monitor hoof health in new animals coming into the flock*
- → *Avoid driving routes, pastures and buildings used by foot rot affected flocks*
- → *Use protective vaccination*
- → *Set up hoof dips*

Foot abscess

Main symptoms

- → *Lameness*
- → *Hypersensitivity to pain*

General: A foot abscess is an infection of the corium caused by various bacteria. It usually affects only one foot in older, heavy sheep and in rams. The bacteria responsible (which occur naturally in the environment and are prevalent in dirty conditions) colonise the skin of the sole, gaining entry through cracks in the horn and minor injuries to the hoof. Pus builds up underneath the hoof horn before finally erupting as an abscess in the space between the toes.

Symptoms: Affected animals develop severe lameness and hypersensitivity to pain in the infected hoof. The abscess between the toes erupts after around eight days. Unlike foot rot, which progresses slowly within a flock, foot abscess is an acute condition.

Treatment: As in foot rot, antibiotic sprays, ointments or powders are applied topically. If an abscess has not yet erupted, it must be opened surgically by your vet. Treatment by

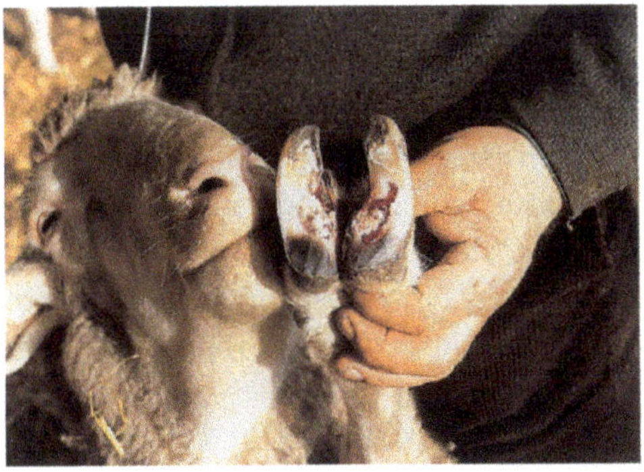

Cauliflower-like growth on both hoof soles

injection of antibiotics has also proved effective. In some cases it may be necessary to bandage the affected hoof.

Preventive measures: Make sure that animals are housed in clean and dry conditions. Hoof dips can help to prevent the disease or stop it from spreading.

Arthritis

Main symptoms

- → *Stiff gait*
- → *Lameness*
- → *Swollen joints*

General: Several bacterial agents cause arthritis, accompanied by lameness and swollen joints, especially in lambs.

Symptoms: Before the age of six weeks, often in association with a navel infection, lambs can develop **acute arthritis** in more than one joint. This disease is caused by several types of bacteria, which gain entry to the body via the navel or minor skin injuries and colonise the joints. The volume of joint fluid increases, accompanied by a swelling or thickening of the joints. Lambs become stiff-legged and go lame. They can develop a high temperature due to the generalised infection.

In older lambs (two to three months old), **chronic arthritis** may be caused by the bacterium ***Erysipelothrix rhusiopathiae*** or by Streptococcus dysgalactiae. The latter also causes erysipelas in pigs. The disease progresses slowly, without fever, and generally without swollen joints. But it is still painful. Lambs show a stiff gait and retarded development. Deterioration of the joint cartilage and bone can cause the joints to become completely locked.

Diagnosis: In both forms of arthritis (acute and chronic), the diagnosis is always confirmed by bacterial culture in the laboratory.

Treatment: Antibiotics should be injected for several days in succession. If the condition has not become chronic, the prospects of recovery are very good. Chronically affected lambs with stiff joints should be isolated and cannot be reared in the flock.

Preventive measures: As a basic principle, wound infections must never be allowed. Navel hygiene and treatment of existing wounds with disinfectant solutions (e.g. iodine) can prevent bacteria from entering the body.

Broken bones (fractures)

Broken bones in the **limbs** are common, but fractures of the **ribs** and **pelvis** also occur. Leg bone fractures are seen in animals in every age group. In lambs, leg bones are often broken by applying traction incorrectly while assisting lambing.

In the case of a **closed fracture** (without an open wound), you can attempt to repair the break using splints or a plaster cast. However, the bones often fail to knit properly. If the animal has an **open fracture** and the wound is infected, the prospects of recovery are poor. Treatment of open fractures is difficult and

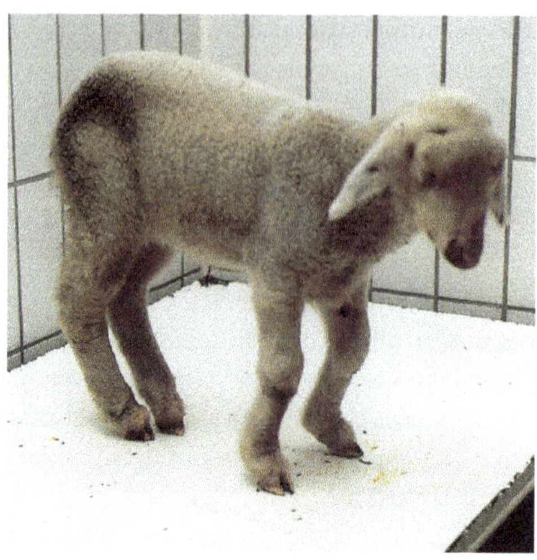

Arthritis: Swollen knee joints in a week-old lamb

should always be undertaken by a veterinary surgeon.

The sheep or goat keeper will consider in each case whether expensive treatment is worthwhile. Veterinary care will be sought for valuable breeding stock.

Contagious ovine digital dermatitis (CODD)

Contagious ovine digital dermatitis (CODD) is the term used to describe a particularly severe form of lameness first reported in the UK in 1997, and now widely reported in the UK sheep sector. The laboratory isolation of spirochaetes resembling those involved in digital dermatitis in cattle from some flocks investigated in detail has led to the adoption of the current name, it was first described as a 'virulent foot rot,' but the foot rot causative organism Dichelobacter nodosus was missing.

The primary lesion in affected sheep begins at the coronary band of the outer wall with subsequent invasion and under-running of the hoof wall from the coronary band towards the toe causing detachment then shedding of the horn capsule (thimbling). Affected sheep are severely lame mainly affecting one digit of one foot in most animals but both digits of one foot in some sheep may be affected and more rarely more than one foot may show lesions. The damage to the corium may be so severe that re-growth of the horn is permanently affected. Typically, there is also loss of hair extending 3–5 cm above the coronary band. There is no interdigital skin involvement.

If the condition occurs during lambing (as in the original outbreak described) – the consequences can be dramatic, as many affected ewes remain recumbent and lambs can't suckle.

Control is based predominantly on keeping infection out, by the application of a sound biosecurity plan developed in consultation with your own veterinary surgeon. The rapid identification of newly lame sheep is an important management practice – the condition can be confused with other forms of lameness, and veterinary advice should be sought before any treatment programme is attempted. Current practice treating foot rot is to move away from conventional foot trimming and removal of under-run horn, to the use of parenteral antibiotic, and this principle should also be applied to CODD control. Both parenteral antibiotic and footbathing affected sheep with antibiotic solutions have been used effectively in early cases (before severe foot pathology has developed).

This condition is the subject of intense veterinary research in the UK, and treatment and control measures may well change as a result. CODD can be spread by hoof knives, so disinfect knives between animals when trimming.

A variant of CODD has been tentatively described in goats in the UK by research workers presenting as severe foot pathology but with solar ulceration as the main clinical sign.

16

Diseases of the respiratory tract

The respiratory tract can be divided into the **upper respiratory tract** (nasal cavity, throat and larynx) and **lower respiratory tract** (trachea, bronchi and right and left lungs with alveoli). The nasal cavity is equipped with sensory cells for the perception of odours. Respiration (breathing) serves to take in and transport oxygen (O_2) and to transport and expel carbon dioxide (CO_2). Oxygen is vital for the body's metabolism. Metabolic processes produce carbon dioxide, a harmful substance that has to be exhaled. Oxygen is taken in and carbon dioxide is excreted via the lungs.

Nasal bot fly

Main symptoms

- *One-sided nasal discharge*
- *Sneezing*
- *Head shaking*

General: The larvae of the **nasal bot fly** or sheep nostril fly *(Oestrus ovis)* cause inflammation of the mucosae (membranes) lining the nose and sinuses. Goats are only rarely affected.

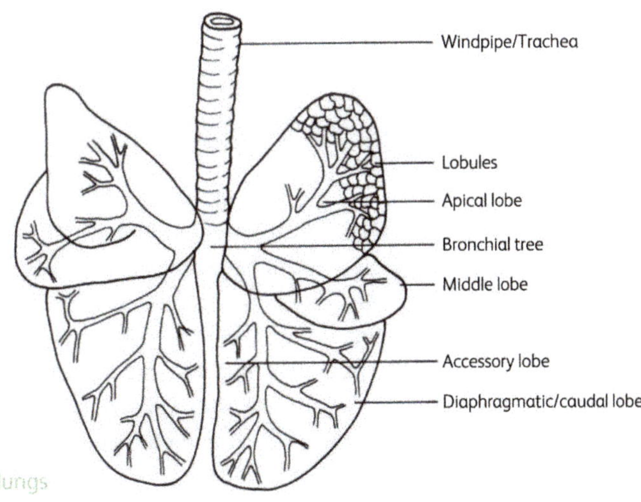

Diagram of the lungs

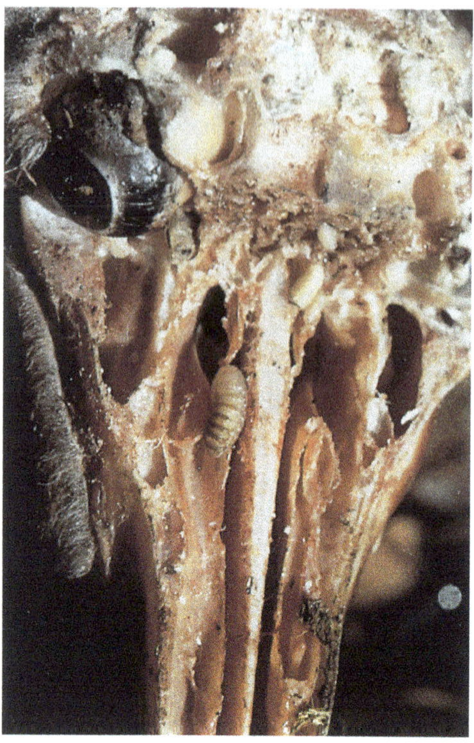

Nasal bot fly larvae in the nasal cavity

The nasal bot fly is a 10–12 mm long, hairy, compact-bodied insect that takes to the wing on warm summer days, usually around midday, and deposits tiny larvae in and around the nostrils of sheep. The larvae make their way into the nose and embed themselves in the mucosae. It is not until the following spring that the larvae develop into the second and third larval stages. These are sneezed out by the host and pupate in the soil, developing into the next generation of adult flies.

Symptoms: The first symptom in sheep infected with nasal bot is a mild nasal discharge. This is clear at first and then changes colour due to secondary bacterial infections. The second and third instar larvae are large and constantly irritate the nasal mucosae, causing sheep to sneeze, hold their noses low to the ground and shake their heads. Animals often have trouble eating and lose weight. Very rarely, the larvae migrate up into the brain, causing meningitis and locomotor disorders.

Diagnosis: The following clinical symptoms suggest a diagnosis of nasal bot infestation:

- Nasal discharge, usually one-sided
- Sneezing
- Nose scratching
- Head shaking

These symptoms almost invariably occur in the spring.

Treatment and preventive measures: Animals in affected areas can be treated orally in the autumn using, a liver flukicide that is also effective in cases of nasal bot infestation. Macrocyclic lactones kill the first instar larvae developing in the nasal cavity. If treatment is delayed and is not given until the second and third instar larvae have developed inside the nose, the killing of these large larvae can have unwanted side effects. There is no way to stop the adult flies from depositing eggs in and around the nose.

If preventive treatment is carried out comprehensively and consistently in the autumn, it may prove possible to eradicate nasal bot infection in endemic areas.

Lungworms

General: Sheep and goats can contract both large and small lungworms. Infection with large lungworms leads to bronchitis and pneumonia, whereas small lungworms rarely cause visible symptoms. At slaughter, small grey pinhead-sized nodules are observed in the lungs of animals with small lungworm (hence the alternative name 'nodular lungworm').

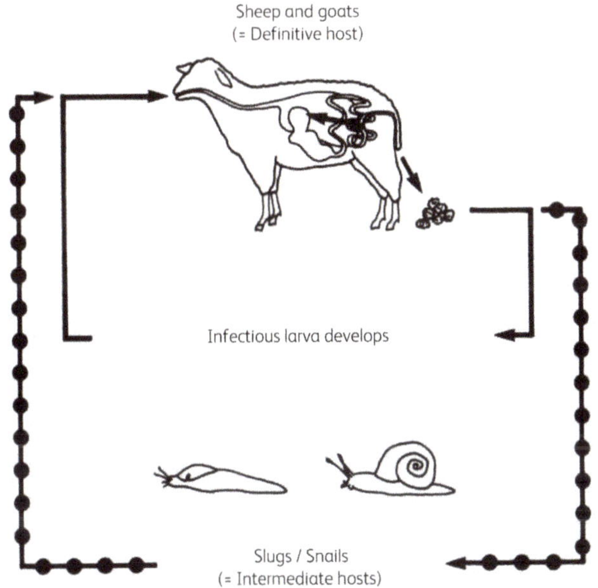

In large lungworm, infectious stages develop directly from the eggs excreted in dung. These stages are swallowed by grazing sheep and goats and then grow into adult worms in the definitive host. In the case of small lungworms, larval development involves an intermediate host (slugs and snails)

*Large lungworm (*Dictyocaulus filaria*)*

Main symptoms

- → *Rapid breathing*
- → *Dry cough*
- → *Nasal discharge*

General: Female worms living in the bronchi of the lungs produce eggs which, after being coughed out and swallowed, end up in the host's gastrointestinal tract. Here, they develop into the next stage (first larval instar), which is excreted in dung. After a week (in summer) to four weeks (autumn), they have developed into the infectious third larval instar, which is ingested by grazing sheep and goats. After migrating from the gut to the lungs, they develop into adult lungworm females, which in turn produce eggs in the bronchi. The interval between infection and detection of lungworm larvae in the dung is 28 days.

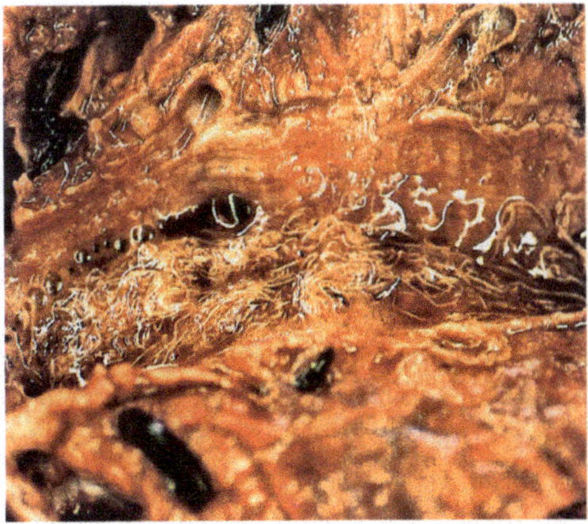

Lungworms in the bronchi and airways cause increased mucus production and inflammation

Symptoms: Around three weeks after infection, animals show rapid breathing, a dry cough and nasal discharge. They usually develop a secondary bacterial infection (pasteurellosis) accompanied by fever, lack of appetite and pneumonia. Weight loss is rapid. Deaths can occur in lambs. If the disease becomes chronic, the animals develop anaemia, poor growth and wool damage.

Goats are more susceptible than sheep and display more pronounced symptoms.

*Small lungworms (*Muellerius capillaris*)*

Main symptoms

- *Isolated bouts of coughing*
- *Non-specific*

General: As with large lungworms, eggs are produced in the lungs. The eggs hatch into first instar larvae that migrate via the airways to the throat. They are then swallowed and excreted after passing through the stomach and intestines. The larvae are very resilient in the outside world. Using slugs and snails as intermediate hosts, they can withstand weeks of frost, overwinter and remain infectious for up two years.

Sheep and goats become infected by swallowing these intermediate hosts while grazing. In the definitive host, the larvae migrate via the gut wall and lymph vessels to the lungs, where they develop into adult worms.

Symptoms: The symptoms that occur following infection are subtle and non-specific, though isolated bouts of coughing may be observed. Here too, goats are more susceptible than sheep.

Diagnosis*: Parasitological examination of dung. **Treatment*:** Large lungworms can be treated with the well-known commercial wormers. Small lungworms are difficult to control with medication because different species respond differently to the drugs available.

Preventive measures*: Regular worming for gastrointestinal parasites using broad-spectrum wormers also reduces lungworm infection rates and the symptoms caused by lungworms. Worming in the spring can prevent the infection from spreading at pasture, as larvae are not excreted during the grazing season. It is not possible to control the slugs and snails, which act as intermediate hosts for small lungworms.

Pulmonary adenomatosis

Main symptoms

- *Clear, almost watery, nasal discharge*

General: This chronic contagious disease of the lungs, also known as Ovine Pulmonary Carcinoma (OPC) or as Jaagsiekte, is caused by a virus belonging to the herpesvirus family and leads to breathing difficulties and weight loss.

Infection: The disease is transmitted by contact with infected animals, which excrete the pathogen via their airways. Lambs contract the infection in the first few weeks of life from their mothers, who remain asymptomatic. The interval between infection and the onset of symptoms is six months to two years.

Symptoms: Infected animals develop rapid breathing, coughing and a clear bilateral nasal discharge, but no fever. Animals

* applies to both large and small lungworms.

hold their heads stretched out. They lose weight and develop bacterial secondary infections in the lungs.

Diagnosis: A clear, almost watery, nasal discharge is the most obvious symptom in the live animal. This can be assessed by conducting a 'wheelbarrow test', in which the animal's hind legs are lifted above the level of its head. This should only be briefly performed before euthanasia as a diagnostic aid – it can be very stressful for the sheep. The low, outstretched head position allows clear discharge to flow freely from the nostrils. The wheelbarrow test is only useful once around two thirds of the lung are already damaged and the virus has therefore been circulating in the flock for some time. Bronchoalveolar lavage with PCR examination allows an early diagnosis.

However, a diagnosis of pulmonary adenomatosis is normally confirmed by post mortem examination in a veterinary testing facility. Typical signs of neoplastic (tumour-like) growth can be seen on examining affected lung tissue under the microscope.

Treatment and preventive measures: This disease generally goes unnoticed in a flock until advanced lung damage has already occurred. As a result, treatment is difficult and the chances of success are low.

Trials to eradicate the disease through motherless lamb rearing have been carried out at the University of Veterinary Medicine in Hannover, with a degree of success.

However, this eradication method is labour-intensive and usually not feasible in a roaming flock. In this case, early identification and removal of affected animals are necessary in order to prevent the virus from spreading. By taking consistent measures like these, it is possible to keep animal losses under control and eventually, after several years, to achieve a largely disease-free flock.

Other types of pneumonia

Combined infections with Staphylococci, Streptococci, Mycoplasmas and possibly Chlamydiae can also cause pneumonia. Fungal infections of the lungs are rare in sheep and goats in Europe. Coughing, laboured breathing, weight loss and fever are typical symptoms. The veterinary surgeon will identify the cause of pneumonia by examining sick or dead animals.

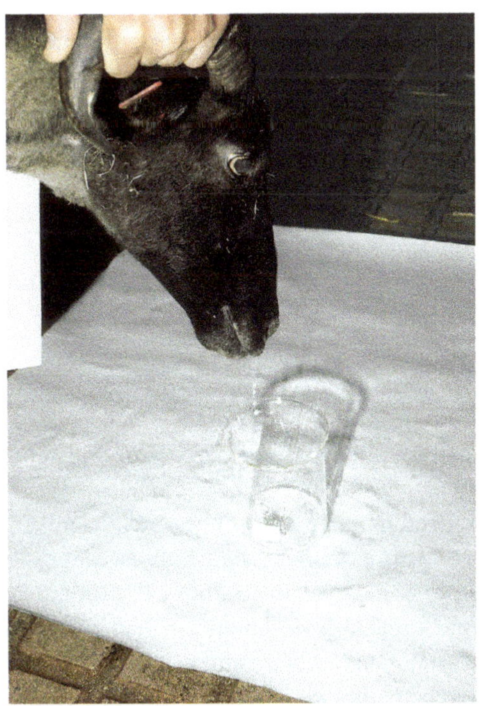

In pulmonary adenomatosis, the 'wheelbarrow test' causes a clear, watery mucous discharge to flow from the nostrils

17

Diseases of the digestive organs

The digestive tract extends from the mouth to the anus and can be divided into four portions:

- mouth, throat;
- oesophagus, forestomachs, abomasum;
- small intestine;
- large intestine, caecum, rectum and anus.

The **mouth** and teeth are used to break down and swallow food, and to perceive taste. The **oesophagus** connects the mouth and forestomachs. In the **forestomachs** (rumen, reticulum and omasum), the feed is broken down, mixed and digested. Indigestible crude fibre (cellulose) in the food is fermented and broken down by bacteria and infusoria (rumen microorganisms). Rumination (chewing the cud) returns the food to the mouth where it is broken down further. Once the cud has been re-swallowed and water extracted in the omasum, the food bolus is transported to the **abomasum.**

Here, it is broken down further with the aid of enzymes.

In lambs, the forestomachs are small and inactive. The milk flows through the 'oesophageal groove' directly into the abomasum, where it is processed. As the lamb begins to eat fodder, the forestomachs enlarge and become active.

The actual process of digestion by pancreatic enzymes takes place in the **small intestine**. The nutrients are broken down into small building blocks, which are absorbed by the lining of the gut and conveyed via the bloodstream to the liver. Here, they are either stored or converted into substances for the body's own use.

In the **large intestine**, cellulose is processed further by bacteria, resulting in fermentation and decomposition processes.

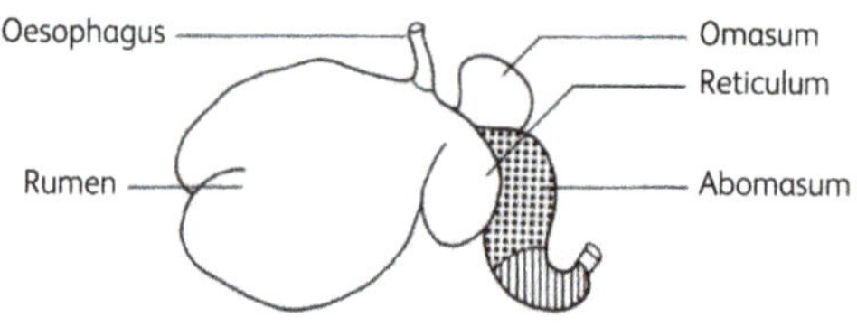

Diagram of the ruminant stomachs.

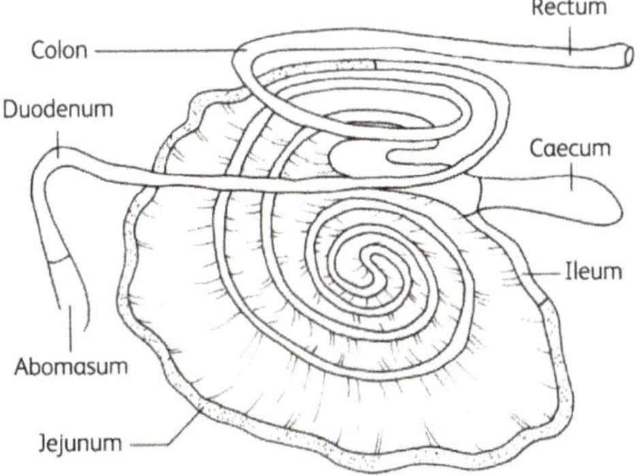

Diagram of the ruminant gastrointestinal tract

Water absorption thickens the remaining food bolus, producing faeces.

The passage of food through the forestomachs, abomasum and intestines is controlled by the autonomic nervous system.

Mouth, teeth

Necrotising stomatitis also known as diphtheria

Main symptoms

- ➔ *Ulcers in the mouth*
- ➔ *Fever*

General: This disease causes inflammation and ulceration of the mouth and throat, destroying the mucous membranes. It usually occurs as a result of Orf infection **Fusobacteria** *(Fusobacterium necrophorum).* The bacteria can also penetrate the mucosae through minor injuries in the mouth caused by sharp grasses or cereal husks.

Symptoms: The disease most commonly affects **suckling lambs**. Lambs stop suckling, become lethargic and develop a fever (40°C). Large ulcers covered with a yellowish coating are seen in the mouth. Due to poor milk intake, lambs lose weight quickly, weaken and die.

Diagnosis: Based on clinical picture.

Treatment: Treatment is unsuccessful in lambs with advanced disease. Milder cases can be treated topically with astringent pastes. Administering penicillin, e.g. using mastitis tubes, has also proved effective. Injection of suitable antibiotics is the optimal treatment.

Note: To prevent infection and to stop Fusobacteria from spreading, it is vital to pay attention to hygiene and cleanliness. If lambs are being reared separate from their mothers, drinking buckets and rubber teats should be cleaned and disinfected regularly.

Conditions of the teeth

Main symptoms

- ➔ *Poor feeding*
- ➔ *Weight loss*
- ➔ *Tooth abnormalities*

General: Diseases of the teeth are almost always confined to the individual animal. Infected teeth or misalignments (including of the back teeth) accompanied by irregular wear can occasionally be observed in older sheep. Foreign bodies (e.g. fodder, wire) getting stuck between the teeth can cause infection.

Symptoms: In affected sheep, tooth disease leads to poor feeding due to a loss of chewing and ruminating ability. Animals lose weight despite an ample supply of feed, and prefer softer types of fodder. Tooth abnormalities can be identified by careful examination of the teeth and mouth.

Treatment: Individual infected teeth can be removed by your veterinary surgeon.

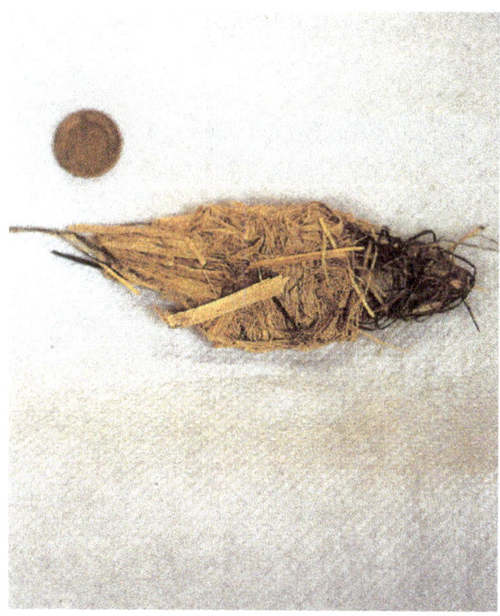

Compressed straw can damage the lining of the mouth

Disinfectant solutions such as tincture of iodine are used to treat the site of infection. Misalignment of entire rows of teeth causing irregular wear cannot be corrected or treated.

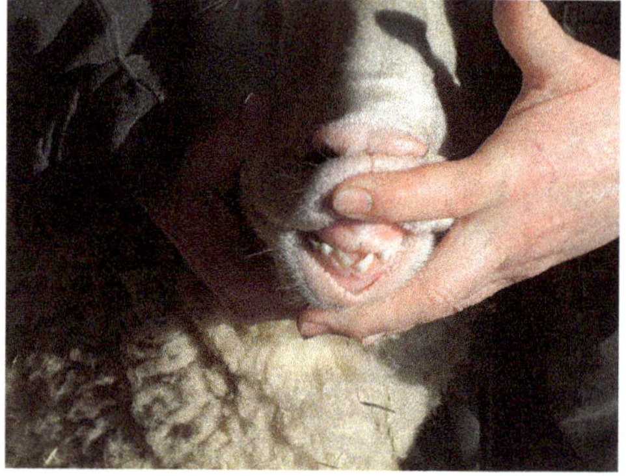

Misalignment of the lower teeth

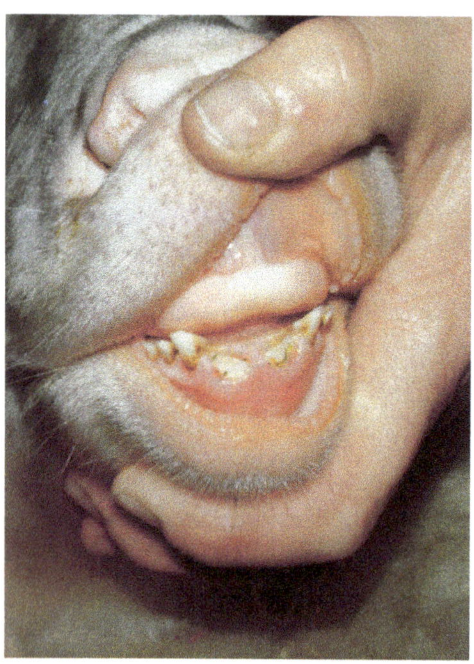

Normal tooth eruption in the sheep

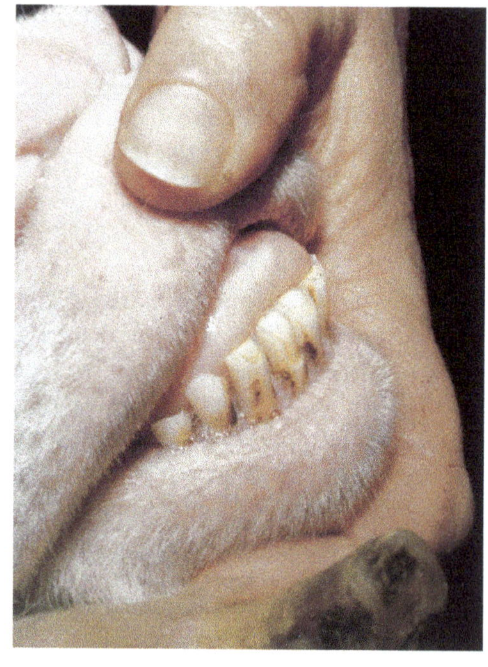

Diagonal wear on the incisors due to tooth misalignment

Forestomachs and abomasum

Rumen acidosis

Main symptoms

- → *Flock-wide disease after eating carbohydrate-rich food*
- → *Convulsions*
- → *Lack of rumen activity*
- → *Stiff gait*
- → *'Downer' animals*

General: Over-consumption of carbohydrate-rich feeds (cereals, sugar beet, beet leaves with heads, potatoes, maize, fruit, bread) in sheep unused to such feeds causes rumen pH to fall below 6 (i.e. become acidic). This can lead to a serious impairment of overall health, sometimes accompanied by high mortality in the flock.

Large quantities of carbohydrate-rich feed cause increased production of lactic acid in the rumen. The body is unable to break down these high levels of lactic acid. Rumen pH (normally 6.2 to 7.0) can become acidified, dropping as low as 4.0. This changes the bacterial composition of the rumen, restricting digestive activity.

High acidity obstructs the movements of the rumen and can even bring it to a complete standstill. At the same time, fluid is extracted from the blood ('blood thickening') and lactic acid levels rise in the bloodstream.

These changes in the rumen and the blood cause severe symptoms in sheep. Symptoms can appear within as little as three to six hours after eating carbohydrate-rich feed. There are two influencing factors:

1. Low water intake before eating accelerates the symptoms, i.e. drinking enough water slows down the rapid acidification.
2. Gradually getting animals used to carbohydrate-rich feed helps to prevent severe symptoms.

Symptoms: In sheep, the disease usually affects the whole flock. Depending on the quantity of carbohydrate-rich feed consumed, the symptoms can range from mild, temporary disorders to serious generalised conditions.

In the **temporary form**, a stiff gait, short-term lack of appetite and mild lethargy can be observed.

In the **severe form** (large quantities of carbohydrate-rich feed without prior habituation) the sheep become lethargic, refuse food and water, and grind their teeth. Rapid breathing and convulsions are observed. Rumen movements come to a standstill and pressing on the flank causes pain. Animals become stiff and ultimately 'go down', ending up completely unable to move, with legs stretched out from the body.

Diagnosis: Post-mortem examination of animals in a veterinary institute reveals a very full rumen. The contents smell sour and have a pH below 5 although pH measurements at PM are of dubious value. Undigested quantities of feed remain in the forestomachs.

Treatment: The veterinary surgeon will treat individual animals with digestion enhancers, fluids and appropriate drugs to neutralise the excess acid in the rumen and restore normal rumen function.

If the whole flock is affected, drinking water should be provided immediately. However, water should be taken to the flock rather than vice-versa because driving the sheep to water would aggravate the symptoms. Chalk can be added to the water to neutralise the acidic pH in the rumen. The diet should consist of good-quality hay.

Acutely affected animals in severe pain should be euthanased.

Preventive measures: Get animals gradually accustomed to carbohydrate-rich feed: if keeping animals on cereal stubble or sugar beet, start with 10 to 20 minutes per day, increasing to two hours over the course of 8 to 10 days. Before grazing such areas or feeding carbohydrate-rich feed, animals should be well watered and fed a fibre-rich diet (hay, old grass).

Rumen alkalosis

Main symptoms

- *Protein-rich feeding*
- *Lack of rumen activity*
- *Swaying*
- *'Downer' animals*

General: Excess dietary protein increases the production of ammonia (a degradation product of protein metabolism) in the rumen, causing the pH to rise to 7.5/8.0. The bacteria and single-celled organisms in the rumen are unable to process excessive amounts of ammonia. This results in overloading of the liver, which is not able to eliminate toxins from the body.

Symptoms: The disease usually affects fairly large numbers of animals. Sheep stop eating, and rumen activity and rumination come to a standstill. Thin, foul-smelling diarrhoea is sometimes observed. Animals sway on their feet and 'go down'.

Diagnosis: Analysis of rumen fluid. It is important to know what the animals have been eating in order to rule out other digestive disorders (such as acidosis).

Treatment and preventive measures: The first step is to stop feeding protein-rich feed. In **mild cases**, this is often enough. In **acute cases**, you can administer solutions that return the high rumen pH to normal levels. After the initial treatment – and once the diagnosis has been confirmed by analysis of rumen fluid – the bacterial rumen flora can be returned to normal by administering fresh, body-temperature rumen fluid from healthy animals (obtained from the slaughterhouse). The veterinary surgeon should administer treatment to protect the damaged liver.

Note: After withdrawing the protein-rich feed, it is important to maintain a diet of good-quality hay and a little beet pulp.

Ruminal bloat

Main symptoms

- *Distended left flank*
- *Rigid posture*

General: Gassy Bloat – gas accumulates form in the upper part of the rumen due to an inability to expel gas produced during fermentation ('belch'). This can happen if the oesophagus is obstructed, e.g. by food residues such as pieces of beet. The resulting gases collect in the upper part of the rumen.

'Frothy' bloat is caused by eating certain foodstuffs such as lucerne, clover, rapeseed, beet leaves or frozen fodder. These bind the gases in a froth of small, stable bubbles which cannot be expelled.

Symptoms: Both gas bloat and frothy bloat are characterised by a marked distension of the left flank. Animals become immobile and rigid. Without treatment, the condition leads to digestive disorders accompanied by collapse with animals lying on their sides. Ruminal gas bloat tends to be a disease of individual animals (oesophageal obstruction) whereas frothy bloat affects the whole flock because usually all of the animals have eaten the feed responsible.

Treatment and preventive measures: If only one animal is affected, the veterinary surgeon should use a probe to check if the oesophagus is clear. Foreign bodies (pieces of feed) should be removed. The veterinary surgeon will inject antispasmodics to support the animal's recovery.

If frothy bloat is affecting a large proportion of the flock, the feed responsible should be withdrawn immediately. Drugs to reduce bubble surface tension should be administered. If such drugs are not immediately available, you can also try using a drench to reduce surface tension.

Once the symptoms have abated, the animals should be fed a diet rich in roughage.

Intestinal parasites

Coccidia

Main symptoms

- → *Watery, foul-smelling diarrhoea with traces of blood and mucus*

General: Coccidia are single-celled parasites that occur in sheep and goats. They are microscopic organisms that live in the intestinal mucosae, where they replicate, initially asexually and then sexually. Outside the body, the permanent form of the organism – the spherical or oval oocyst – can survive for several months in cold weather. In warm and humid conditions, however, spores mature within the oocysts. The spores are infectious, so the disease (**coccidiosis**) can develop once they have been swallowed with feed.

Coccidia occur in many species of animal but are highly host-specific. This means that the species of Coccidia found in sheep and goats are not passed on to other animals.

Nowadays, coccidiosis tends to be a disease of indoor animals, especially fattening lambs. But it also occurs in lambs kept on pasture.

Infection: The main source of infection is adult sheep which are carrying and shedding Coccidia. Lambs are particularly susceptible, becoming infected via direct ingestion of mature oocysts in feed contaminated with dung, through contact with dirty bedding or by swallowing pathogens clinging to the dam's udder. Damp, dark buildings with dung-contaminated piles of feed, feed containers and drinkers, high stocking densities, mixing of age groups and small paddocks increase the risk of infection. Lambs between 6 and 12 weeks old are especially prone to infection and disease if the dam has a poor milk supply and they are not receiving enough additional feeding.

Coccidiosis is influenced by weather, temperature and humidity on the one hand and by husbandry conditions and the animals' resilience to disease on the other.

Symptoms: The first symptoms are observed in lambs between four and seven weeks old. In animals kept at pasture, the disease peaks and losses occur in May/June. In motherless rearing with cold milk

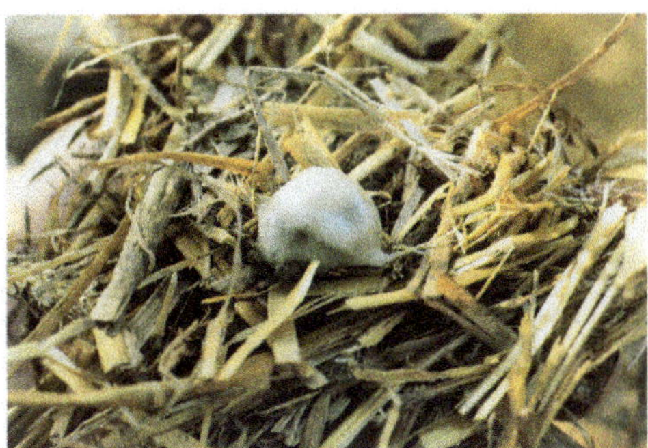

Droppings coated with mucus are typical of Coccidia infestation

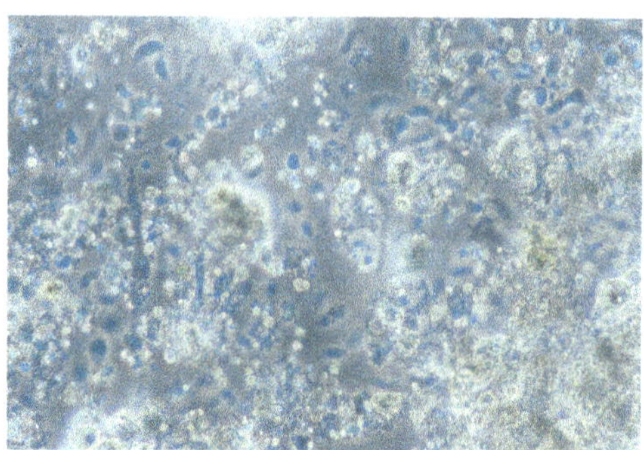

Detection of oocysts by parasitological examination of dung

feeding, faecal testing of lambs detects coccidial oocysts as early as day 13; with warm milk feeding, oocysts are detected by day 20. The first sign of disease is droppings coated with threads of mucus, resembling a string of pearls. Typically, the main symptom is watery, foul-smelling diarrhoea, which can be greenish or blood-tinged. The consequences include soiling of the fleece around the back end, lethargy, anorexia and obvious weight loss.

Severe intestinal bleeding can occur in acute cases. Mass outbreaks lead to deaths among the lambs within a few days. In less aggressive cases, the infection progresses more slowly and anaemia and wasting are observed in addition to diarrhoea. Lambs can recover but their development is retarded.

Diagnosis: Faecal testing for oocysts can be carried out in the laboratory or veterinary practice and gives a quick, reliable diagnosis.

Treatment: Affected lambs should be housed in small groups with dry, fresh bedding and clean feed troughs. Lambs should be checked daily. A suitable diet consists of good-quality hay and easily digestible feedstuffs.

Drug treatment should be given under veterinary supervision. Treatment consists of special anticoccidial products. Wormers are **not** suitable: Coccidia are not worms but single-celled organisms and have a completely different metabolism.

Preventive measures: It is vital to promote disease resilience in the animals and to reduce the risk of infection. A balanced diet including minerals and vitamins, plus regular control of worm diseases, helps to prevent a weakened immune system.

Clean drinkers, troughs and mangers, dry bedding and the avoidance of ground feeding all reduce the risk of coccidial infection.

Note: It is impossible to prevent sheep and goats from becoming infected with Coccidia. However, in order to avoid losing animals, it is important to strike a balance between disease resilience and levels of coccidial infection. Resilient animals generally cope well with coccidial infection. Prevention using drugs is recommended only if all other precautions have failed or cannot be put in place.

Special disinfectants can kill coccidial oocysts in buildings and on troughs and drinkers. Always follow the manufacturer's instructions.

Gastrointestinal roundworms (nematodes)

Main symptoms

- → *Diarrhoea*
- → *Weight loss*
- → *Lack of energy*
- → *Anaemia*
- → *White mucous membranes*
- → *Throat swelling*

General: Gastrointestinal worms include various species of roundworm which occur at different sites in the bodies of sheep and goats and can be transmitted between them. The diseases caused by these roundworms are of considerable economic importance in sheep and goat keeping.

Worm development and infection: To carry out targeted control of roundworm infestations, you need to know how long it takes the parasites to develop, both inside the animal's body and outside it on pasture. All roundworms have basically similar developmental cycles.

The worm eggs excreted by sheep and goats contain a first stage larva which then develops into a third stage larva in the droppings. This process is influenced by temperature and humidity. The third stage larva

Gastrointestinal worms in sheep and goats.

Worm species	Pathogenicity	Development on pasture	Development in the animal (prepatent period)
Abomasal worms			
Haemonchus contortus (barber's pole worm)	+++		
Teladorsagia sp. (brown stomach worm)	+++	6 days, can overwinter	3–4 weeks
Small intestinal worms			
Trichostrongylus sp. (hairworms)	++	6 days	3 weeks
Cooperia curticei (roundworms)	+	5 days	2–3 weeks
Nematodirus filicollis (hairworms)	++	can overwinter in the egg, otherwise 3 weeks	3–4 weeks
Bunostomum trigocephalum (hookworm)	+++	around 3 weeks	2 months
Strongyloides sp. (threadworm)	+	4 days	1 week
Large intestinal worms			
Oesophagostomum venulasum (large bowel worm)	+	7 days	around 3 months
Chabertia sp. (large–mouthed bowel worm)	+	7 days	(1) 3–5 months
Trichuris sp. (whipworm)	+	around 3 months	2 months
Tapeworms			
Moniezia expansa	+	4–5 months	4 weeks
Moniezia benedeni	+	4–5 months	4 weeks
+++ high ++ moderate	+ low		

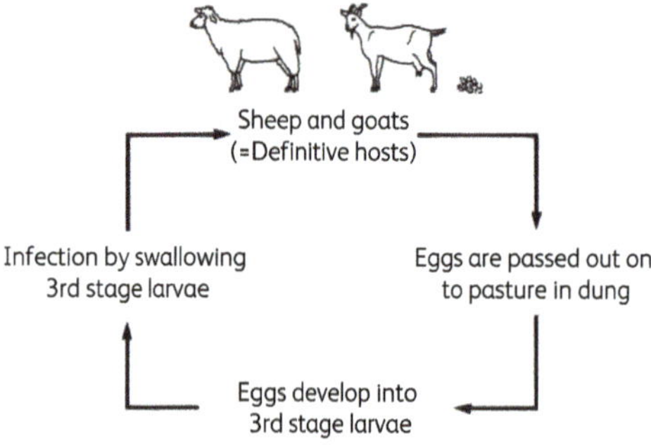

Developmental cycle of gastrointestinal nematodes (roundworms) of sheep and goats. Larvae hatch from the eggs excreted in dung and are then swallowed by grazing animals

can be detected in drops of dew. It climbs up blades of grass and is swallowed by grazing sheep and goats. This is the start of its development inside the animal, which ends with the sexually mature worm. Male and female worms mate, and the females start to lay eggs which in turn are excreted in the dung. The interval between the ingestion of the third stage larvae and the excretion of new worm eggs in dung is called the **prepatent period.** During this period, no eggs are detected in the dung despite the presence of infestation.

Regarding development inside the animal, it should be noted that barber's pole worm, brown stomach worm, hairworms, large bowel worm and large-mouthed bowel worm can all undergo a period of dormancy inside the host. This can extend their development to several months, i.e. these worms overwinter in the gastrointestinal mucosae of sheep and goats. In the case of hookworms and threadworms, the infectious larvae penetrate the skin and migrate via the bloodstream to the lungs, and only then to the gut. In the spring, and just before and after lambing, ewes shed huge numbers of worm eggs, leading to massive contamination of spring pastures and thus to a higher risk of infection for the lambs. This is another important factor to consider when controlling worm infestations.

Symptoms: The **abomasal worms** *Haemonchus contortus* and *Teladorsagia* spp. damage the mucosal lining of the abomasum. *Haemonchus* is a blood-sucking parasite (consuming around 15 ml per 1000 worms per day). Goats are highly susceptible, especially to *Teladorsagia* infection. The resulting blood loss causes anaemia, pale mucous membranes, lethargy and poor weight gain or weight loss. Infestation with small and large intestinal worms (usually combined with abomasal worm infestations) is accompanied by diarrhoea, poor feed utilisation and emaciation. No diarrhoea does not mean no worm infestation! 'Bottle jaw' (throat oedema) develops in animals with a heavy worm burden. This symptom is not indicative of a particular worm disease (e.g. liver fluke).

The best way to assess an animal's weight loss is to feel along its back: normally the muscles should cover the bones comfortably.

The symptoms of worm infestation are especially clear in lambs. Older sheep have often built up a good immunity. However, this immunity can break down due to poor husbandry and feeding, or under a severe parasite burden.

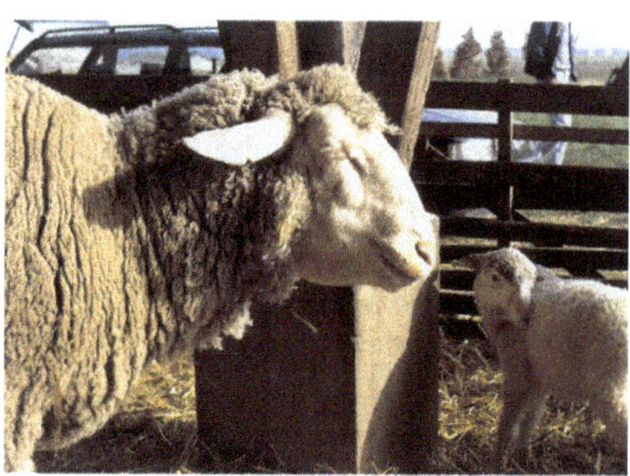

Typical 'bottle jaw' in a sheep with a heavy worm burden

Infection, egg shedding, disease caused by gastrointestinal roundworms.

Worm species	*Infection in spring on pasture*		*Egg shedding (lambs)*	*Infection*	*Disease*
	Overwintering stages	*Dams after lambing*			
Barber's pole worm *Haemonchus contortus*	–	+++	July	July	from July
Brown stomach worm *(Teladorsagia)*	++	+++	June	June	July to autumn
Hairworm *(Trichostrongylus sp.)*	+	+	June	June	Autumn
Hairworm *(Nematodirus sp.)*	Larva in egg	–	May to June	May in the following year	May

+++ high ++ moderate + low

In such cases, adult sheep too will show emaciation and pale mucous membranes, and sometimes diarrhoea.

Diagnosis: Faecal testing.

Treatment and preventive measures: Benzimidazole-resistant species now occur worldwide and their prevalence is on the increase. The parasites have also developed significant resistance to wormers from other active ingredient groups in other European countries and further afield. In South America, for example, there are already certain regions where sheep can no longer be farmed due to the resistance situation. Resistance to new wormers is already emerging. The search for alternative treatment strategies and new methods, possibly biological ones, should be a top priority in the future. Such alternatives are already beginning to take shape but are not yet ready for use in practice, e.g. the feeding of sheep and goats with fodder plants containing tannins, or the addition to feed of fungal spores which, after passing through the animal, kill worm larvae in its droppings. **Causes of resistance** include:

- frequent use of wormers from the same active ingredient group (benzimidazoles);
- under-dosing;
- parasites with primary resistance 'surviving' treatment.

The **barber's pole worm** and **brown stomach worm** *(Haemonchus, Teladorsagia)* and small intestinal hairworms *(Trichostrongylus, Nematodirus)* are already showing such resistance.

Worming programmes for sheep and goats should therefore take account of worm resistance and also consider the individual pasture situation of each flock.

A **worming programme** that includes tapeworms aims to interrupt the development of the worm population in various locations:

- on infected pastures,
- in buildings,
- in the host animal.

A selection of preparations for parasite control in sheep and goats (without liability).

Preparation		*Efficacy against*							*Withdrawal period (days)*		*Notes*
	Active ingredient	Gastro-intestinal worms	Small lung-worms	Large lung-worms	Tape-worms	Liver fluke	Coccidia	External parasites	Meat	Milk	
Benzimidazoles											
	Mebendazole	+	(+)	+	(+)				7		Not in dairy sheep, ideally not in pregnant sheep
	Mebendazole	+	(+)	+	(+)				7		Not in dairy sheep, ideally not in pregnant sheep
	Fenbendazole	+	(+)	+	(+)				10	3	Tapeworms 2 ml/kg bodyweight
	Fenbendazole	+	(+)	+	(+)				21	3	
	Oxfendazole	+	(+)	+					14	5	Not in dairy sheep
	Albendazole	+	(+)	+	(+)	+			12	5	Large liver fluke: 5 ml/10 kg
	Triclabendazole	+	(+)	+	(+)	+			28	12	Not in dairy sheep and first-time mothers 2 months before lambing
Levamisoles											(Follow dosages in this group precisely)
	Levamisole	+	(+)	+					21		Not in dairy sheep
	Levamisole	+	(+)	+					8		Not in dairy sheep
Macrocyclic lactones											
	Moxidectin	+	+	+					14	5	
	Ivermectin 0.5/25	+	+	+					42		Not in dairy sheep

Combined preparations									
	Moxidectin, triclabendazole	+	+		+		31		Not in dairy sheep and pregnant animals 2 months before lambing
	Closantel, mebendazole	+	+	+	+				Not in dairy sheep
Other									
	Praziquantel			+			0	0	
	Closantel	(+)			+		42		Not in dairy sheep
	Diclazuril					+	0		Licensed only for lambs and sheep
	Toltrazuril					+	42		Not in dairy sheep
	Monepantel	+				+	7		No resistance currently known

Follow the manufacturers' withdrawal periods for meat, milk and organs. Work with your vet tɔ devise a treatment plan for your flock that takes account of wormer resistance. Compiled and updated by Dr. Johannes Winkelmann, Kiel.

+++ excellent
++ good
+ moderate
* effective at higher doses per animal
** effective only against barber's pole worm; + to ++ also against immature liver fluke *** effective only against adult fluke

General recommendations:

- Faecal sample monitoring: Which parasites are present?
- No changes of pasture.
- Follow-up monitoring: repeat faecal sample testing 7 to 10 days after treatment.
- Dosages: adapt wormer dosages to the maximum weight of the animals to be treated.
- Dosing device: check its accuracy.
- Avoid changing wormers within an active ingredient group.
- Preventing the introduction of resistant worm species: quarantining new animals, worming, post-treatment monitoring.
- Keeping animals healthy, slowing development of resistance in parasites.

Worming: Your aim should be to keep your animals healthy and to slow the development of the parasites' resistance. To this end, within a group of sheep or goats, you should worm only the animals that are visibly affected: emaciation, diarrhoea, pale mucous membranes. Sheep can transmit resistant worms to goats, and vice versa. Goats should be treated with a higher wormer dosage than sheep.

Worming should be combined with appropriate **pasture hygiene**:

- Pastures are 'clean' in the spring, if they are freshly sown, ungrazed (mown only), or grazed by horses only in the previous grazing season.
- Pastures are 'low risk' if they are used for hay.
- Pastures are 'high risk' if they were grazed by lambs and yearlings in the previous year.

Using available pasture land to produce hay also reduces a pasture's worm burden.

These measures are all aimed at slowing down the spread of resistant worm species. If keepers know their animals well and monitor them carefully, they can adopt **further recommendations** which also reduce the risk of resistance:

- Lambs should be protected against disease by regular worming. However, they must be allowed to build up immunity, i.e. if the lambs are healthy and well-developed, the intervals between treatments can be lengthened (NB: regular monitoring of the animals' health is vital).
- Treat dams less often (but monitor them carefully). Worming animals before feeding improves the efficacy of the product.

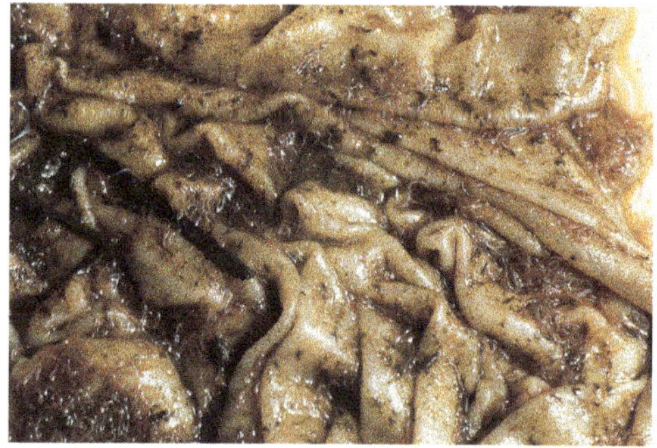

Worms in the opened abomasum of a dead sheep

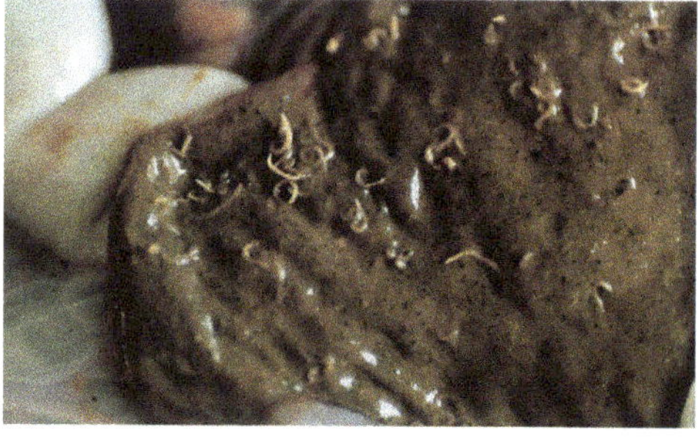

Worms in the opened large intestine of a dead sheep

Targeted selective treatment: Worming and pasture hygiene taking account of farm conditions (pasture/paddock keeping, roaming flocks, dairying, etc.) help to avoid high losses due to parasitic diseases and to slow down the development of resistant parasites.

Note: Parasitological tests to establish the parasite burden should be carried out just before each scheduled treatment. Treatment can then be carried out if necessary. Follow-up tests are carried out a week after treatment.

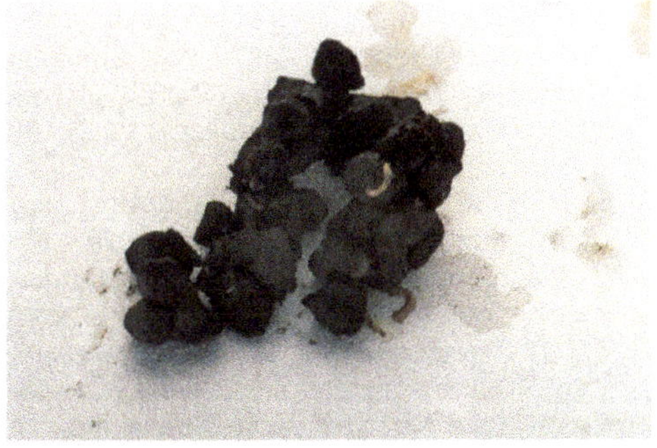

White tapeworm segments are clearly visible in dung

Tapeworms

> *Main symptoms in lambs*
>
> → *Distended bellies*
> → *Stretching*
> → *Tapeworm segments in dung*

General: Two important species of tapeworm that occur in sheep can also be transmitted to other ruminants, including goats, and from the latter to sheep. They are *Moniezia expansa* und *Moniezia benedeni.*

Worm development and infection: Sheep tapeworms require moss or pasture mites (Oribatida) as an intermediate host in their developmental cycle. Moss mites occur on pasture, and indoors in old bedding. The mites eat tapeworm eggs excreted by the sheep. Inside the mite, the eggs develop over a period of four to five months and hatch into the infectious intermediate form of the parasite, which sheep and goats then swallow together with the mite. The intermediate form can also overwinter in the mite. After being swallowed by the sheep or goat, the parasite develops over six to eight weeks into the adult tapeworm, which can survive in the animal for 3 to 8 months.

Symptoms: Tapeworm infestation generally affects lambs (two to four months old). Symptoms include distended bellies, colic-like pain, stretching and weight loss. Emaciation and fertility problems are observed in adult sheep. However, tapeworm infestations in older animals are often asymptomatic. As the first symptoms appear, tapeworm segments start to be excreted in batches and can be detected in the dung.

But worm segments are not necessarily spotted first: an infestation can be present without visible evidence.

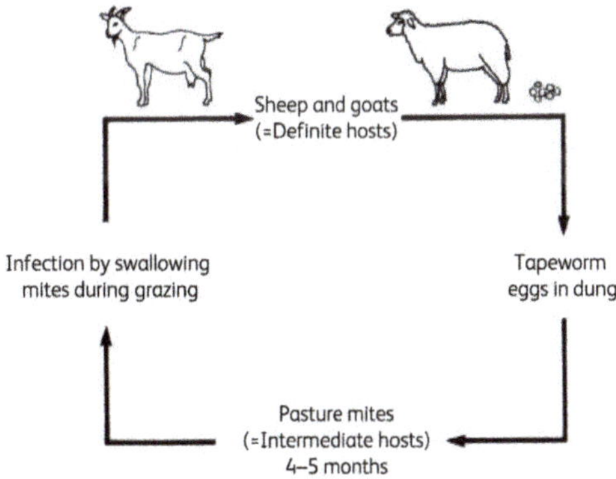

Developmental cycle of the sheep and goat tapeworm *Moniezia expansa*. Tiny pasture mites act as an intermediate host

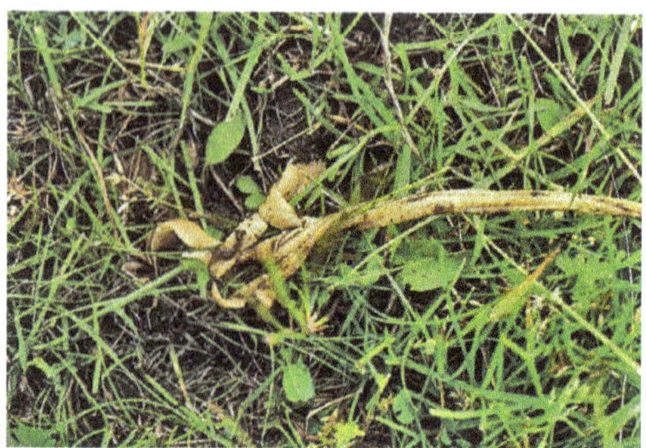

Excreted tapeworm segments on pasture following treatment

Treatment: Sheep are treated for tapeworm in May. If tapeworm segments appear again in the dung, treatment can be repeated in the summer or autumn. To prevent contamination of pastures, sheep should be kept indoors for around two days after worming.

Preventive measures: The intermediate host (pasture mites) cannot be controlled. Old bedding should be removed from buildings regularly to prevent tapeworm infestation.

Tapeworm cysts

General: Sheep and goats are intermediate hosts to three species of tapeworm that occur in dogs and foxes (the definitive hosts). An intermediate larval stage of the tapeworm, called a cyst, develops inside the sheep or goat.

Cyst development and infection:

1. The **sheep measles cyst** *(Cysticercus ovis)* takes the form of a small, fluid-filled sac or 'bladder', which attaches to the peritoneum or omentum in the abdominal cavity. The cyst is the larval stage of the tapeworm *Taenia ovis,* whose final hosts include dogs and foxes. Sheep and goats swallow the tapeworm eggs when grazing fodder plants contaminated with dog or fox faeces, and they then serve as cyst carriers.
2. The **gidworm cyst** *(Coenurus cerebralis)* lodges in the brain and is the larval stage of the dog or fox tapeworm *Taenia multiceps.* Here too, sheep and goats swallow the tapeworm eggs as they graze.
3. The **Echinococcus cyst** *(Echinococcus hydatidosus),* which occurs in the liver, is rarely seen in sheep and goats. It is the larval stage of the dog and fox tapeworm *Echinococcus granulosus,* which in this stage also poses a risk to human health.

Symptoms: There are no noticeable symptoms. Only the gidworm causes visible symptoms, due to its location in the brain.

Diagnosis: The sheep measles cyst and Echinococcus liver cyst are generally not detected until slaughter.

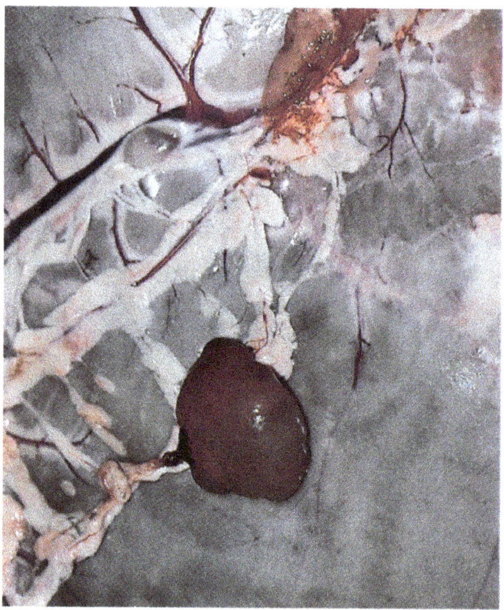

A sheep measles cyst in the rumen – a chance finding on post mortem. The sheep had not been displaying any symptoms

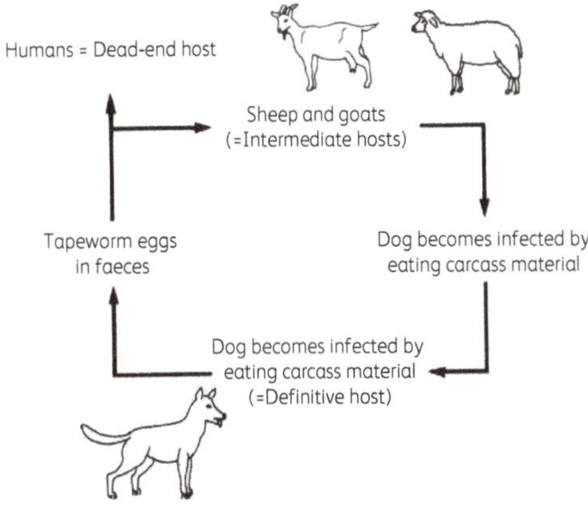

Transmission route of the dog and fox tapeworm *(Echinococcus granulosus)*

Treatment: Drug treatment can be attempted for affected sheep and goats but is justified only in the case of valuable breeding animals, and the results are dubious.

Preventive measures: The most important measures are regular faecal testing for dogs and appropriate worming. Dogs should be kept away from the flock for two days after worming, until the tapeworm segments and eggs have been excreted. It is also important not to feed animal carcasses or uncooked slaughterhouse waste to dogs, especially herding dogs. If possible, pet dogs should be kept away from pastures used for sheep and goats. However, this may be difficult to achieve in practice.

Johne's disease (paratuberculosis)

General: Johne's disease is a chronic infection of the large intestine caused by *Mycobacterium avium* sp. *paratuberculosis* (MAP). In the UK it is a serious problem in the commercial goat sector, and is not uncommon in the sheep sector. Besides affecting sheep and goats, it also occurs in cattle. However, different subtypes of Mycobacterium are found in each of the three species of ruminant. The possibility of cross-infection is currently being investigated and is a subject of controversy (do sheep and goats contract the infection from cattle, or vice versa?). MAP bacteria are also found in wild ruminants, rabbits and several species of bird.

However, this disease is of particular importance in connection with **Crohn's disease** in humans, as the pathogen *M. paratuberculosis* has also been detected in people with Crohn's. This raises the question of what the relationship might be between the infection in domestic ruminants and the disease in humans. Much remains to be explained in this respect, and assumptions and speculation should be avoided until the outstanding questions have finally been resolved.

The disease in cattle, sheep and goats is observed more frequently in certain regions with acidic pasture soils.

Infection: Mycobacteria are ingested from the soil by grazing animals and then harboured in the digestive tract. Animals without symptoms can also shed the pathogens. Lambs are thought to become infected in the uterus (although this has not yet been demonstrated) or via milk and contact with the dung of infected dams.

Symptoms: Usually, no symptoms are observed, even in infected sheep and goats. Clinical signs encountered can be severe though, in the absence of any other concurrent problem. An outbreak can occur if the disease burden is especially high, e.g. due to other pathogens such as parasites, Pasteurella, etc. The most common symptoms are emaciation despite a good appetite and loose, watery diarrhoea that does not respond to treatment. Diarrhoea however is a feature of the disease in cattle, whereas in sheep and goats it is not until the terminal stages. Animals die or have to be euthanased due to the progressive, severe emaciation.

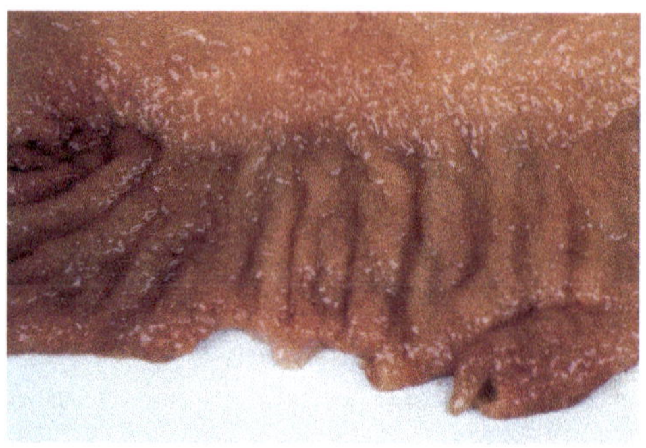

'Brain-like' thickening of the ileal mucosa caused by Johne's disease

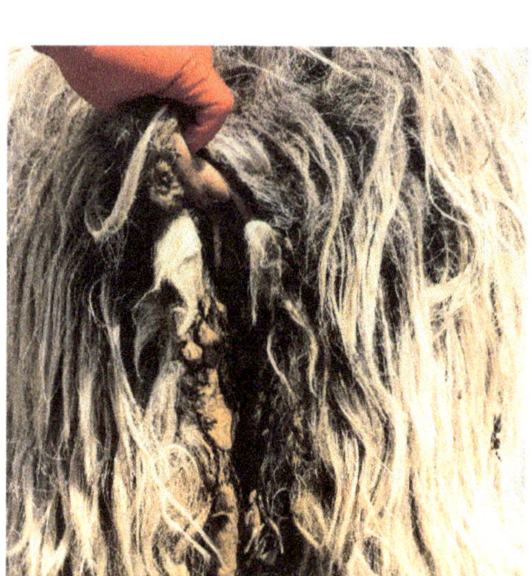

Uncontrollable loose, watery diarrhoea is a symptom of Johne's disease

Diagnosis: On post mortem, a thickening of the gut wall can be seen in individual sections of the large and small intestine. The typical acid-resistant Mycobacteria are found on microscopic examination. A diagnosis can also be obtained by conducting a blood test. Blood testing can also serve as a potential basis for control.

Treatment: In the UK there are many control measures that can be put in place, including a vaccine and test and cull programmes.

18

Diseases of the liver

The liver is the body's most important metabolic organ. In the liver, nutrients absorbed in the intestines from food are converted into substances that the body can use (protein, carbohydrates, fats). Glycogen, fats, vitamins, iron, copper and zinc are stored in the liver. At the same time, the liver detoxifies the blood passing through it. It produces bile, which the body needs in order to digest fat. Lastly, the liver acts as a blood store and plays a role in the body's immune defences.

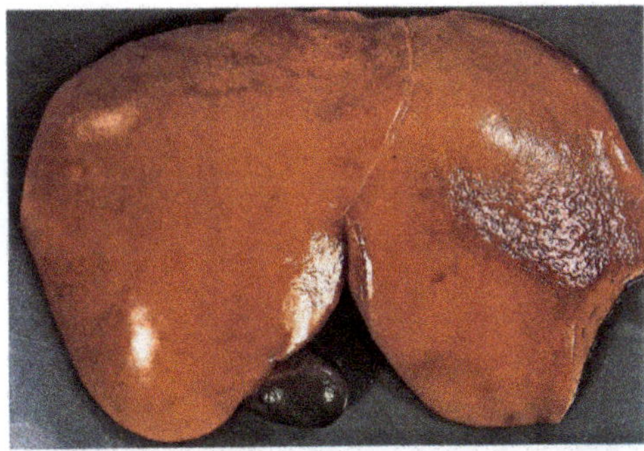

The brownish-yellow discolouration of this liver points to copper poisoning

Liver fluke disease (fasciolosis)

Main symptoms

- → *Weight loss*
- → *Anaemia*
- → *Jaundice, usually in the autumn*
- → *Poor wool quality*

General: Liver fluke occurs in Central Europe in cattle, sheep, goats, roe deer, red deer, fallow deer and occasionally in horses. It colonises the liver's bile ducts, leading to a disruption of liver metabolism.

Liver fluke development and infection: Adult flukes in the bile ducts lay eggs which pass into the small intestine and from there to the large intestine before being excreted onto the pasture with the animal's dung. In temperatures above 10°C, the fluke egg hatches into a mobile larval stage with cilia (a 'miracidium'). This swims about in ponds and puddles in search of its intermediate host, the dwarf pond snail, and penetrates its body. Another mobile form (a 'cercaria'), this time with a tail, develops within the snail. After leaving the snail, it settles on plants in the pasture. The infectious permanent forms of the parasite ('metacercariae') are then swallowed by grazing sheep or goats. In the host's intestine, these hatch into immature flukes which burrow through the intestinal wall, penetrate the liver and ultimately migrate to the bile ducts, closing the cycle. The time between ingestion of the metacercariae and the laying of eggs in the bile ducts is 56 days in sheep and 65 days in goats. The developmental period can also be longer, depending on the animal's general state of health.

Symptoms: In sheep and goats, the subacute form of the disease (during the migratory stage of the immature fluke) is the most significant stage, with the clearest symptoms. Animals go off their food and quickly lose weight. They develop anaemia, jaundice, ascites and peritonitis; pregnant animals abort. Symptoms are usually observed in the autumn (September).

In the chronic form, which occurs in the winter, typical symptoms include emaciation, poor fertility and reduced wool quality. The animals' general condition is poor.

Treatment and preventive measures: There are three ways to control liver fluke disease:

1. Eliminating the intermediate host

The dwarf pond snail, which acts as an intermediate host, lives in shallow fresh water in areas with high groundwater tables and impermeable alkaline soils. Banks of streams, ditches and rivers provide an ideal habitat for the snail. From there, they can also colonise wet pasture land, hollows and watering holes. Pasture management measures such

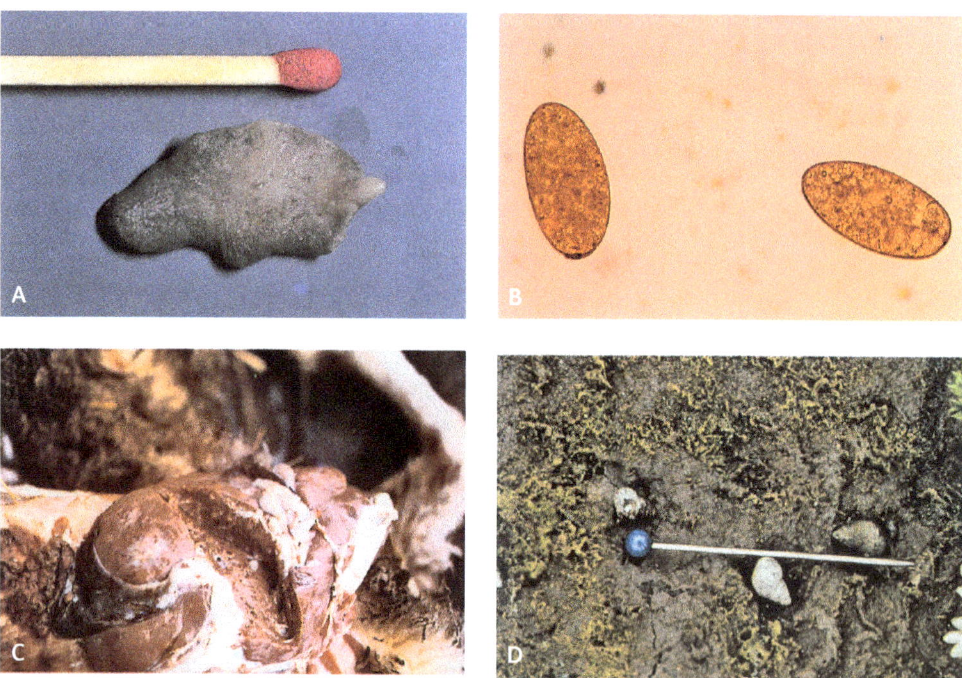

The liver fluke (a) settles in the bile ducts and lays its characteristic eggs (b) which are passed out with the dung. A liver destroyed by liver fluke (c). The snail used by liver fluke as an intermediate host is barely larger than a pinhead (d)

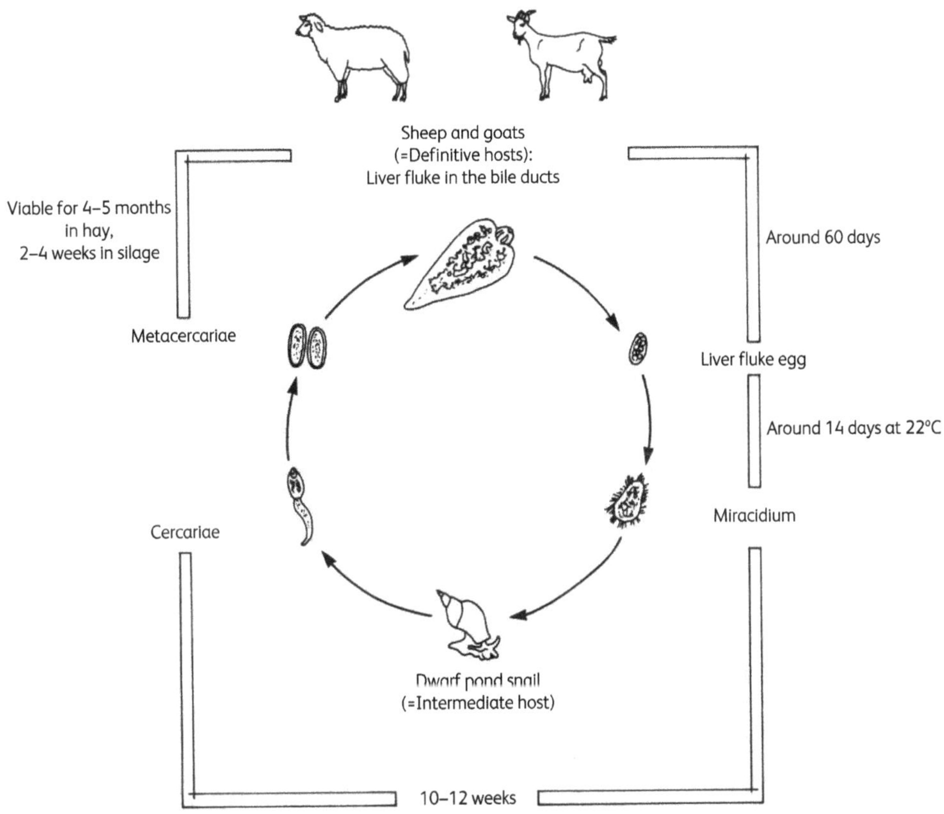

Developmental cycle of the common liver fluke (*Fasciola hepatica*). A free-swimming miradicium hatches out of the egg and enters the body of a dwarf pond snail, the intermediate host. Several stages of development occur in the snail, resulting in large numbers of cercariae, which are then released from the snail. The next stage is the permanent form (metacercariae), which settles on blades of grass and remains viable for periods in hay and silage. After the metacercariae have been swallowed during grazing, new liver flukes develop in the sheep or goat

as fencing off damp areas or river banks and draining new pastures can help to eliminate the snail and interrupt the liver fluke's life cycle. Snail control on pasture using molluscicides (e.g. snail pellets) is now rejected on ecological grounds. However, ducks make excellent snail predators and coexist happily with sheep.

2. Preventing ingestion of the permanent forms (metacercariae)

By fencing off river banks and damp, low-lying areas of pasture, and by using troughs rather than watering holes, sheep and goats can be prevented from swallowing the metacercariae as they graze, thus preventing reinfection.

3. Using drugs to treat sheep and goats infected with liver fluke

If subacute liver fluke disease occurs in the autumn (September), treat all animals in the flock with a flukicide that will also kill the immature stage. A change of pasture is essential. Treat again around four to six weeks (October/December) after bringing the animals in from pasture. To prevent pasture contamination, a further treatment should be carried out before turning them out again (March/April). If the autumn was wet, treat again in the following August because overwintered snails can release metacercariae in the spring. This means that the cycle has not been interrupted and animals can become reinfected.

Necrobacillosis

General: In various diseases such as navel ill, foot rot and Orf, inflammation and ulceration are caused by bacteria spreading via the bloodstream or – as in navel ill – migrating to the liver. Scattered abscesses develop in the liver, sometimes growing to the size of a walnut. Necrobacillosis is usually confined to individual lambs.

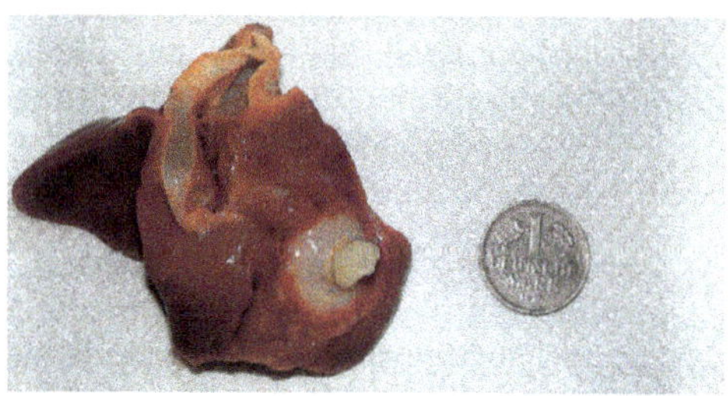

Pus-filled abscesses in a lamb's liver (coin Ø 23.5 mm)

Symptoms: The abscesses in the liver are hard to diagnose. This is because, as in the case of spreading navel ill, there are rarely any clear symptoms. Common signs are a loss of appetite and willingness to suckle, lethargy and tight, strained flanks. Animals die within a few days.

Diagnosis: Pus-filled abscesses are found in the liver on post mortem.

Treatment: There is no known successful treatment. If a definite diagnosis has been made, antibiotic therapy can be attempted in the early stages of the disease.

Preventive measures: It is important to avoid navel ill by disinfecting navels and to treat hooves regularly to control foot rot. Local Orf treatment can also help to minimise the spread of the bacteria responsible. Bacteria in the animals' environment can be suppressed by proper cleaning and disinfection of buildings.

19

Diseases of the urinary organs

The urinary organs are closely associated with the reproductive system. In male animals the sperm ducts lead to the urethra; in female animals the urethra ends inside the vulva. The urinary organs include the kidneys, ureters, bladder and urethra. The kidneys and reproductive organs are closely related in both male and female animals.

The functions of the kidney are to excrete toxins and waste substances, to regulate the body's water metabolism and to produce urine. The ureters, bladder and urethra convey the urine out of the body.

The two kidneys filter waste from the blood and excrete around 3–5 litres of urine per day. Urine collects in the bladder, which is emptied by the micturition reflex. The urethra ends and seals the urinary tract.

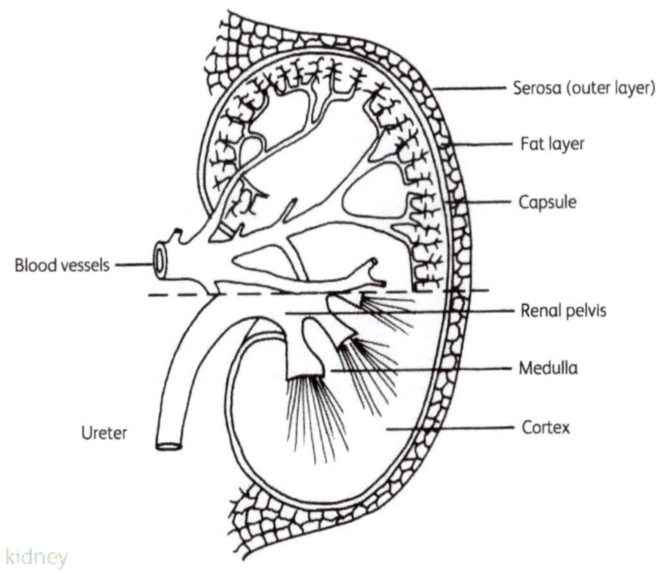

Diagram of the kidney

Urinary stones and sediment (*Urolithiasis*)

Main symptoms

- → *Urinary dribbling*
- → *Unsuccessful attempts to urinate*
- → *Teeth grinding*

General: Urinary stones and sediment ('gravel') occur almost exclusively in male animals and lead to urethral obstruction and urinary blockage.

The disease primarily affects fattening animals on a high-phosphorus, low-calcium diet based on grain concentrates. The increased supply of phosphorus excreted by the kidneys causes crystals of sediment to form in the bladder. These crystals grow into stones, which can obstruct the urethra and block the passing of urine. Other factors involved are a lack of drinking water, transport stress and moving of animals. Merinos are more susceptible than other breeds of sheep.

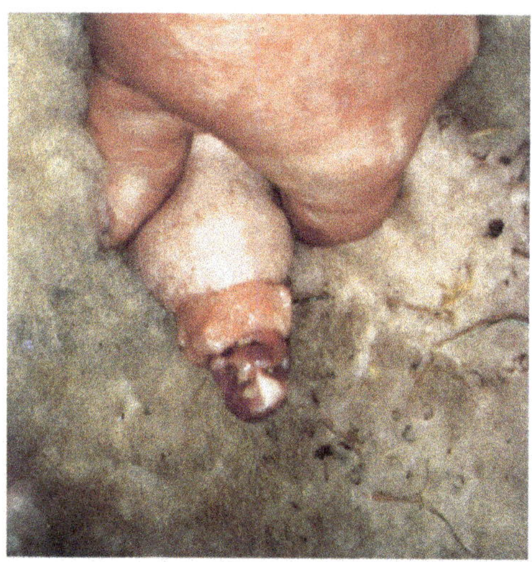

A swollen, inflamed penis tip

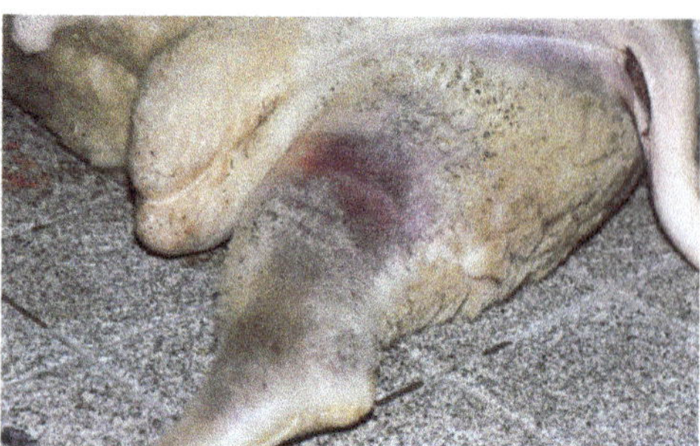

Watery swelling of the inner thigh in a downer animal with chronic urinary obstruction

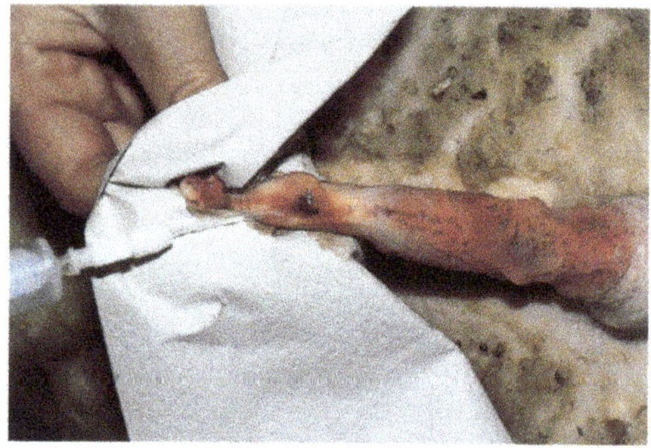

To allow urine flow, the vet attempts to catheterise via a lateral incision in the urethra

Symptoms: A blockage of the urethra due to urinary stones normally occurs at the tip of the penis or in the S-shaped curve (perineal region). Animals go off their food and make repeated unsuccessful attempts to urinate. There may be audible signs of pain such as teeth grinding or groaning. Urine is passed in dribbles; in advanced stages of the disease the animal's breath smells of urine. The belly becomes swollen with fluid ('water belly'). Animals spend a lot of time lying down. If the bladder ruptures the animal may appear to improve temporarily but will die within a day or so.

Treatment and preventive measures: If the stones lodge near the end of the urethra, the tip of the penis can be amputated to allow urine flow. If the stones are further up the urinary tract, the vet can open the urethra surgically and create an artificial opening. However, the prospects of successful treatment are not good. Euthanasia is recommended if the animal's overall condition is poor. Carcasses are unsuitable for human consumption due to the taint of urine.

In the finishing period, provide a Ca/P ratio of around 3:1. Make sure the animals drink enough water. Drinking can be encouraged by providing mineral licks. Adding cattle salt to the animals' concentrates will increase water intake, helping to flush out urinary sediment.

Inflammation of the prepuce

Main symptoms

- *Purulent discharge from the prepuce*

General: Older wethers have a longer foreskin (or 'prepuce') which can retain urine after urination. This provides an ideal breeding ground for certain bacteria, which can then replicate and cause infection. Injuries to the foreskin can also become infected if bacteria are involved.

Symptoms: In the initial stages of the infection, a yellowish discharge comes from the preputial opening. As the condition progresses, the discharge becomes purulent, thick and sometimes bloody. Urination becomes difficult. If treatment is not given at this stage, the preputial opening narrows, preventing urination. The animals show signs of pain, swelling of the foreskin and a stiff gait.

Treatment: The first step is to allow urination. After that, the infection can be treated with disinfectant solutions or antibiotic creams (administered by mastitis tube).

Treatment should be continued until the inflammation subsides, after which regular monitoring is necessary. Reducing the protein content of the feed will also help to accelerate recovery. If this step is taken, mild to moderate cases will subside on their own.

Inflammation of the bladder (cystitis)

Main symptoms

- *Straining to urinate*
- *Arched back*
- *Teeth grinding*

General: Bladder inflammation (cystitis) can occur in both male and female animals. Bacterial infections entering the urinary tract from outside are often the cause. Urine flow disorders are common in female animals following compression of the urethra during lambing. Bacteria are then able to colonise the bladder. In males, cystitis can be caused by an inflammation of the foreskin leading to a disruption of urine flow, or by obstruction of the urethra due to urinary stones.

Symptoms: Typical symptoms include straining to urinate accompanied by arching of the back and signs of pain (groaning, teeth grinding). If the kidneys are involved in the disease process, fever and fatigue may also occur.

Diagnosis: Urine testing with detection of bacteria by your vet.

Treatment: Depending on the severity of the disease, it can be treated locally via a catheter or the vet will inject antibiotics.

Kidney diseases

Kidney diseases in sheep and goats generally occur as a result of chronic infections of other organs (lungs, liver), urinary stones, an inflammation of the foreskin or a navel infection. Poisoning (copper, lead) can cause chronic kidney conditions.

As a rule, kidney involvement is not detected until a post mortem is conducted following the animal's death.

Diseases of the reproductive organs

Male reproductive organs

The male reproductive organs consist of two testicles or testes, two epididymes, two spermatic cords with sperm ducts, the reproductive glands (prostate gland, ampullary gland, bulbourethral gland) and the penis with foreskin.

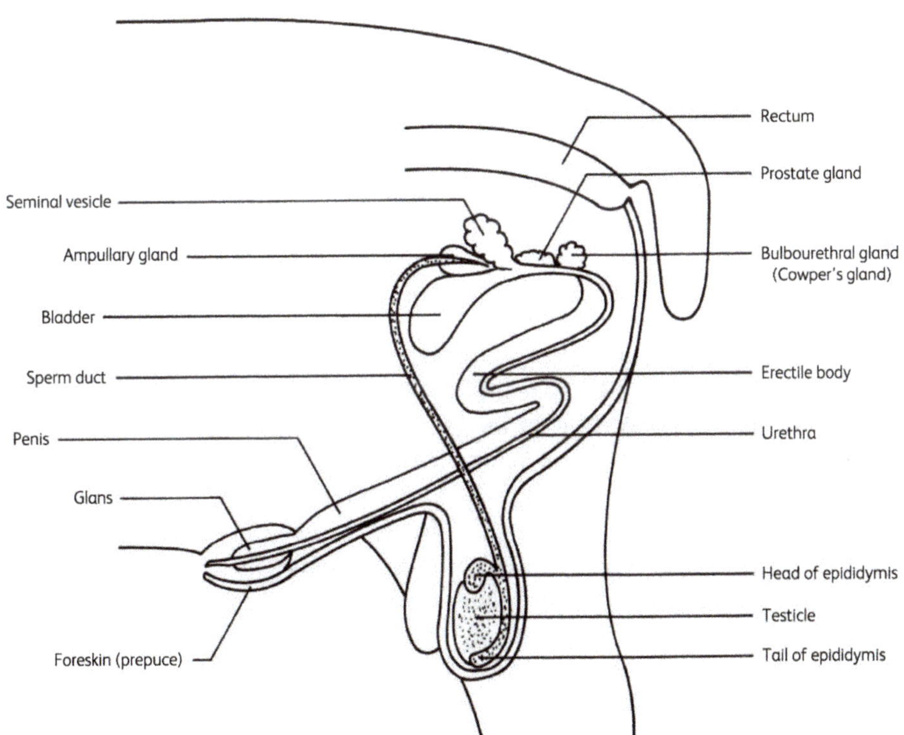

The reproductive organs in the male sheep (von Korn, 2001)

The functions of these organs are to produce sperm (in the testes), to mature sperm (in the epididymes), to produce seminal fluid (in the reproductive glands) and, during mating, to transport the semen to the female reproductive organs where fertilisation occurs. The volume of ejaculate (sperm + seminal fluid) in a ram is 1 to 3 ml, with 3 to 4 million sperm in each ml.

Cryptorchidism

Even before a male lamb is born, both of its testicles should have descended from the abdomen into the scrotum. If only one has descended, the condition is described as **unilateral cryptorchidism**; if neither testicle can be felt in the scrotum, the lamb has **bilateral cryptorchidism**. Testicles that are retained in the abdominal cavity do not produce sperm cells. In unilateral cryptorchidism, the descended testicle does produce sperm cells so the animal has a degree of fertility. If both testicles are retained, the ram is not capable of breeding. Rams with only one testicle are unfit for breeding as cryptorchidism is passed on to the next generation.

Small testicles

This hereditary defect can be congenital (present from birth), in which case it is described as testicular hypoplasia. If the testicles develop normally at first but are found to be small at sexual maturity or later, this is described as testicular atrophy.

Rams with hypoplastic testicles are sterile and incapable of reproducing. Rams with testicular atrophy should be excluded from breeding. Small testicle size can be detected by feeling the testicles within the scrotum.

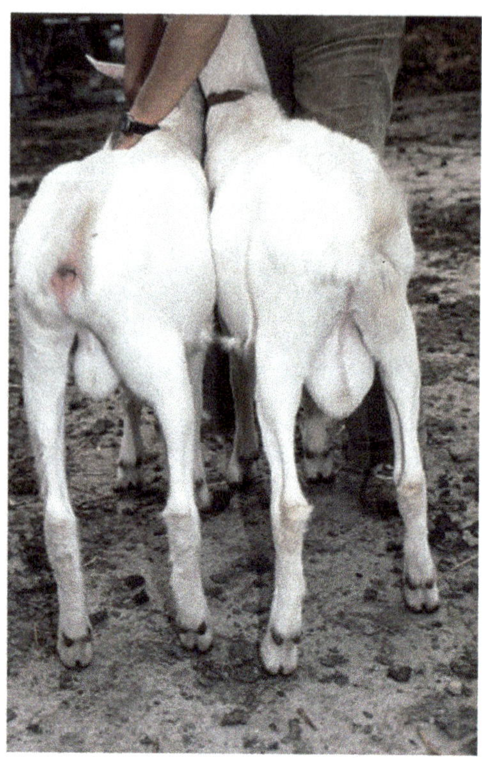

Small testicles in the buck on the left compared with normal development on the right

Testicular inflammation (orchitis)

Main symptoms

- *Testicular enlargement*
- *Hypersensitivity to pain*

General: Testicular inflammation can be caused by an injury (kick, crushing) or by bacterial pathogens.

Symptoms: The testicles become greatly enlarged and bump against the inner thighs as the animal walks. The pain is severe; rams go off their food and are unwilling to move. Affected testicles feel hot to the touch and are very sensitive to pressure.

The animal's mating urge is greatly reduced.

Treatment: Your vet will administer anti-inflammatories or antibiotics.

Note: Remember, brucellosis is a notifiable disease.

Epididymitis

Main symptoms

- Abnormalities can be detected on examination

General: The sperm cells produced in the testicles are matured in the epididymes. Inflammation of these organs (epididymitis) therefore causes fertility problems. Like orchitis (inflammation of the testicles), epididymitis can be caused by pathogens (Brucella, Chlamydia, etc.) or by malformation and injury.

Symptoms: Changes in the epididymes often go unnoticed until the animal has a breeding assessment, e.g. at auction. The two epididymes are compared by feel. An affected epididymis is enlarged and has a nodular structure. Pain is rare. Often, only one epididymis is affected.

Treatment: Not possible. Affected rams are unfit for breeding.

Note: Changes in the testicles and epididymes as described above can severely affect fertility in rams. Because some of these defects (cryptorchidism, small testicles) are thought to be hereditary, affected rams should not be used for breeding.

If orchitis or epididymitis is caused by an infectious disease, a blood test should be conducted to rule out brucellosis, a notifiable disease which is subject to control by the competent Veterinary Office.

Female reproductive organs

The female reproductive organs consist of two ovaries, two oviducts, the uterus, the cervix, the vagina with vaginal vestibule, and the vulva with labia.

After the onset of sexual maturity, eggs are produced in the ovary. On ovulation they are transferred to the oviduct, where they are fertilised by sperm. The resulting foetus implants in the lining of the uterus, where it continues to develop. Signs of oestrus and readiness to mate include restlessness, mounting other animals, swelling of the labia and the production of mucus.

Diseases or abnormalities of the female reproductive organs in sheep or goats tend to be noticed only when the fertility of the flock, or of individual animals, fails to come up to the keeper's expectations. The lambing results for the flock will be calculated, taking into account the results for each dam.

Metritis

Inflammation of the uterus (metritis) can occur as a consequence of an untreated retained afterbirth, after premature births or after injuries sustained during lambing. Retained afterbirths and premature deliveries often have an infectious cause.

If an infection develops, it can extend to the entire abdominal cavity (especially in the case of injuries to the uterus). This can result in a significant impairment of the animal's overall condition, and even in death.

Ringwomb

Narrowing of the vagina often occurs in connection with difficult births and lambing injuries. Scar formation results in narrowing

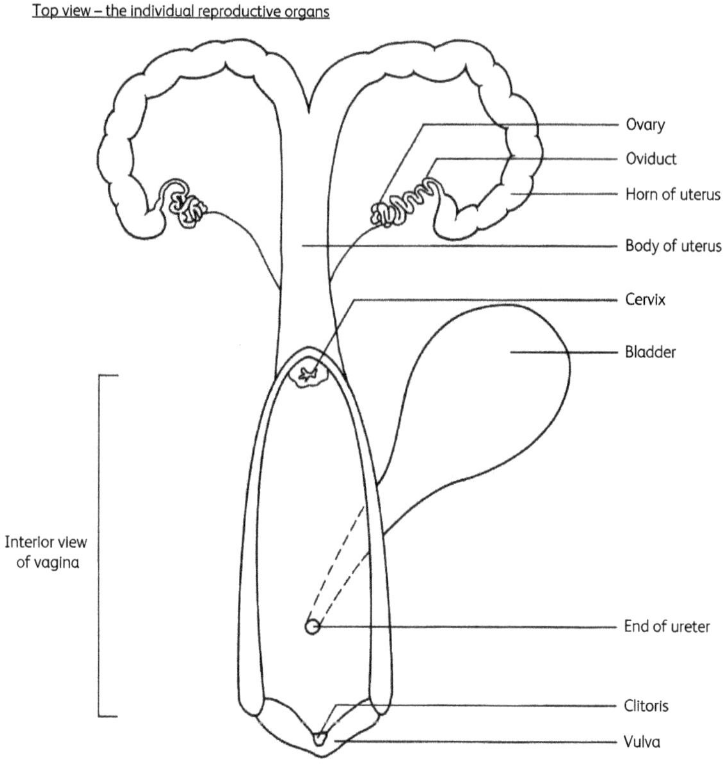

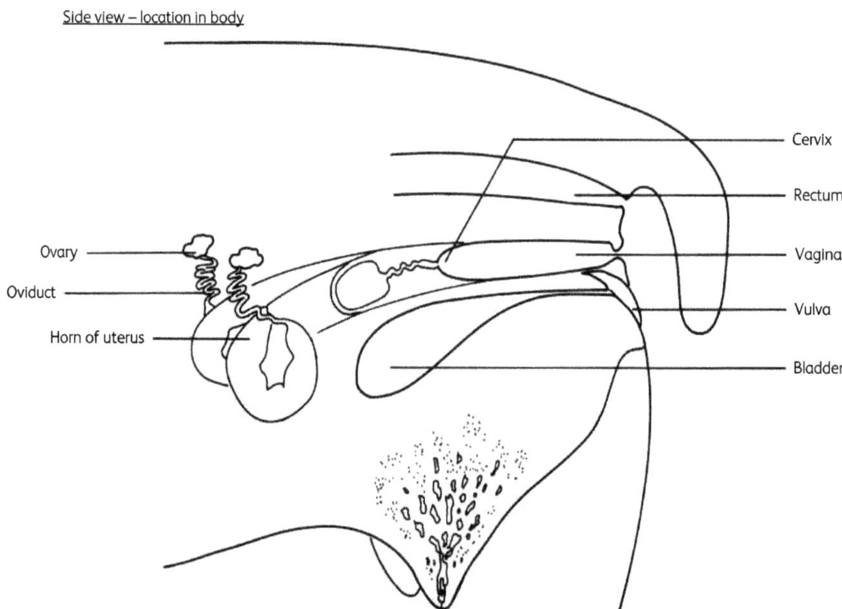

The reproductive organs in the female sheep (von Korn, 2001)

of the birth canal. In these cases, subsequent births will almost always be difficult.

Vulval infections

In the genital form of Orf, the external reproductive organs are also affected. Injuries caused by difficult births and dog bites occasionally occur.

Anoestrus and return to oestrus

Symptoms of fertility problems include anoestrus and return to oestrus. In the case of anoestrus (absence of heat) in young ewes, you can attempt to trigger oestrus by switching to a protein-rich mineral feed or by administering hormone treatment (ask your vet).

If an increased rate of returns to oestrus is observed, specific blood tests can be conducted to rule out infectious causes; it is also important to test the rams used to serve the ewes.

In many cases you will need to consult a vet, who will conduct random testing of individual females and all males in the flock.

Udder

In sheep and goats, the udder consists of two halves. Its function is to produce milk and so to supply the newborns with nutrition. The first milk (colostrum) contains antibodies to protect against diseases, as well as vital nutrients for the lambs.

Suckling and nudging by the lambs causes milk to flow into the milk ducts and teat cisterns.

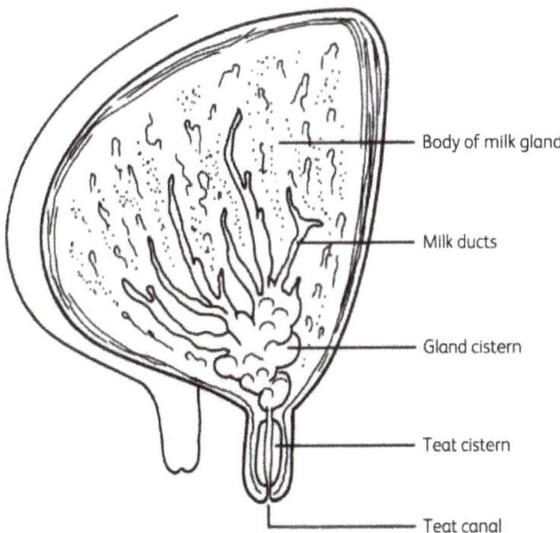

The structure of the milk glands in the sheep (von Korn, 2001)

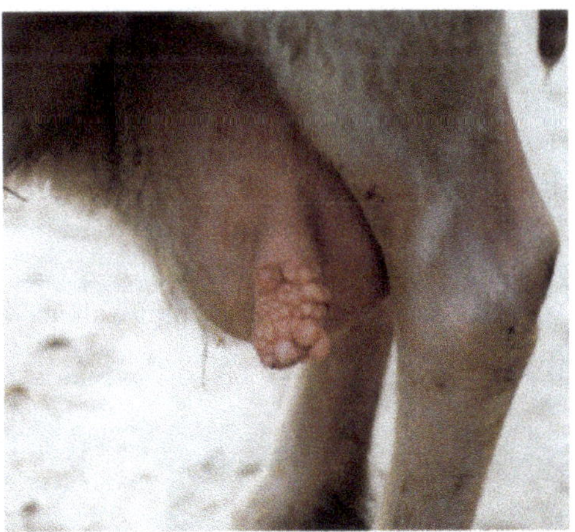

Udder warts make it difficult for lambs to suckle

Udder inflammation (mastitis)

Main symptoms

- *One half of udder is enlarged*
- *Fever*
- *Bluish skin discolouration*

General: Mastitis is an inflammation of one or both halves of the udder. The main cause of acute mastitis is a bacterial infection with *Escherichia coli* and Pasteurella. Infection with *Staphylococcus aureus* tends to cause a chronic condition with scarring in the udder (nodular lesions). These bacteria are present in the animals' surroundings and can enter the milk gland via the teat canal. The teat canal normally forms a barrier against bacteria, but if it is damaged due to injury or crushing (e.g. by older lambs, 'milk bandits') it becomes easier for bacteria to enter. Udder involvement in cases of Orf infection also makes it easier for bacteria to gain access.

Symptoms: Mastitis in sheep and goats usually affects their overall health. Animals adopt a wide-legged stance and kick at the swollen udder with a hind leg. They do not allow their lambs to suckle. Affected animals stop eating and develop a high fever (up to 41°C). The udder is swollen (usually on one side only) and hot, and the skin is discoloured (bluish-black).

Attempts at milking produce only a watery discharge, often mixed with blood.

If mastitis is not spotted promptly, affected animals can die. In other cases, the udder half becomes gangrenous and necrotic, or hard and nodular (lumpy udder).

Treatment: It is important to identify and treat mastitis **promptly**. In the initial stages, your vet will need to inject antibiotics into the muscle in order to bring down the animal's fever and treat its poor overall condition. The inflamed udder should be milked out regularly and intramammary antibiotic tubes used. This treatment should be continued for two to three days until there is a clear improvement. Treatment with antibiotics should also be continued. Rubbing with udder cream supports recovery.

If mastitis is treated early, both udder and dam can be saved. In many cases the animal is saved but the udder becomes useless. If antibiotics have been used, be sure to observe

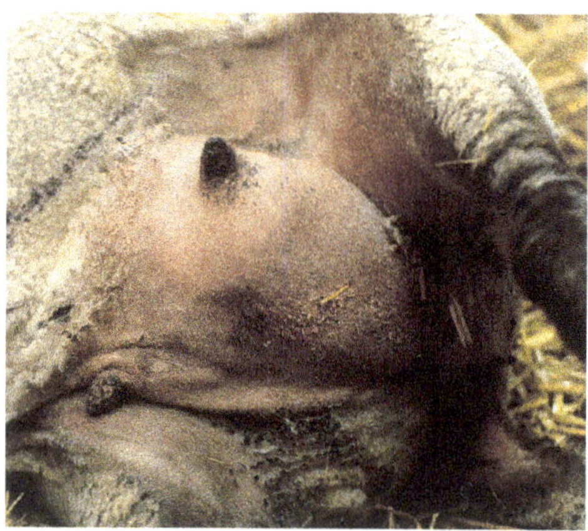

Mastitic udder. The affected half is swollen and reddened. Udder cream has already been applied

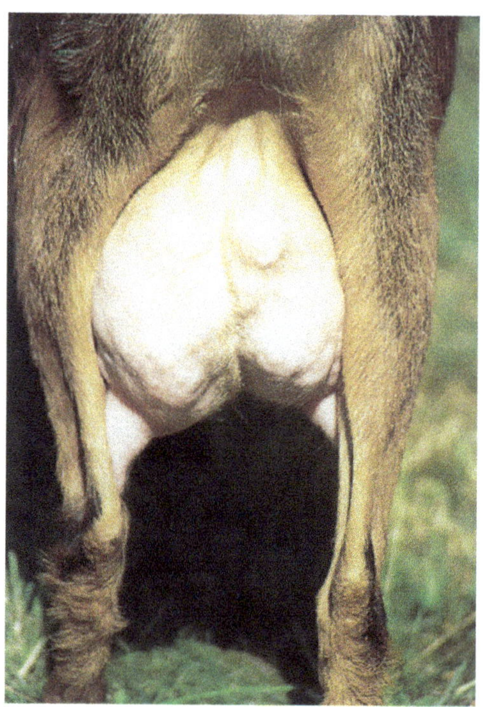

Mastitis: nodules and hardening are clearly visible

the stipulated withdrawal periods before slaughtering animals.

Preventive measures: Building hygiene and clean bedding help to prevent increased bacterial stress on the animals. Milk bandits should be removed from the flock. Once the lambs have been weaned, udders can be protected using 'drying off' products. When administering these, however, take special care to avoid damaging the teat canal.

In dairying operations, regular checks should be carried out to make sure that milking machines are working properly. Teats should be dipped after milking.

Note: Any watery milk or discharge milked off should be collected and disposed of safely. Do not simply milk animals into their bedding as this spreads bacteria.

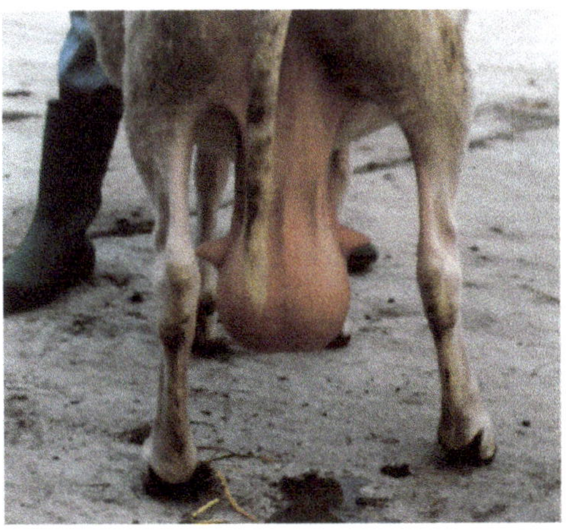

A very low-hanging udder like this is especially prone to injury

Udder and teat Injuries

Udder injuries are often only skin-deep. Injuries can be caused by dog bites, barbed wire and other sharp or pointed objects. Superficial wounds should be cleaned and treated with antiseptics or antibiotics.

Open wounds should be treated surgically by your vet, who will suture them properly. If an individual teat is affected, amputation may be necessary. The udder half should also be surgically removed in order to prevent inflammation.

21

Pregnancy and birth

The development of the embryo takes place in the uterus. Around 14 days after the egg has been fertilised in the oviduct, a permanent connection develops in the uterus between the egg and the mother's bloodstream. Two sets of foetal membranes develop (amnion and chorion or 'water bag'). Their role is to protect the foetus, absorb urine and form the umbilical cord.

The placenta provides sufficient nutrition for the developing lambs in the uterus. Over the course of pregnancy, 150–500 ml of fluid collect in the amnion and up to 1200 ml in the water bag. Ultrasound examination can detect a pregnancy at an early stage based on the presence of fluid in the uterus.

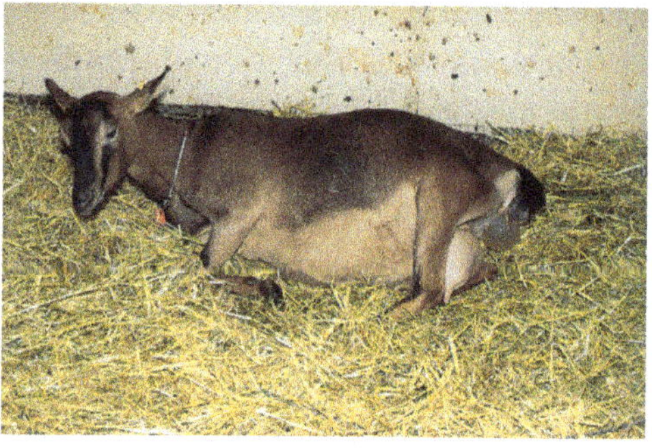

Contractions push the water bag into the birth canal

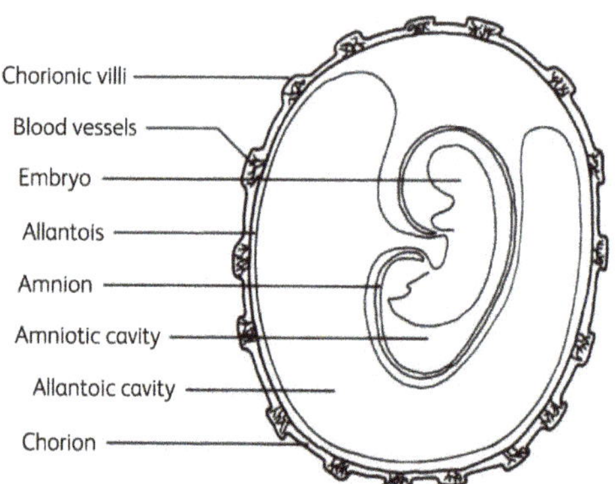

Diagram of the amniotic membranes in ruminants

Contagious causes of abortion

Enzootic abortion (caused by Chlamydophila abortus*)*

Main symptoms

- *Abortion in the last few weeks before birth*
- *Yellowish afterbirth with mucous coating*

General: In pregnant sheep and goats, the bacterial infection can cause abortion, still births and the births of weakly offspring.

Infection: The agents responsible are ingested orally, generally after being shed in massive quantities during abortions (afterbirth, uterine discharge). However, the agents are also shed in milk, urine and dung. Via the bloodstream, Chlamydia bacteria enter the uterus where they cause inflammation, which disrupts the supply of nutrition to the foetuses, which die or become chronically infected. Due to infected lambs and the shedding of bacteria in milk, urine and dung, an infection can persist within a flock for a very long time.

Symptoms: Dams abort in the last few weeks before lambing, without showing any symptoms themselves. Lambs are stillborn or weakly; afterbirths are yellowish, swollen and coated with a slimy, often viscous fluid.

In a first-time infection in a flock, up to 50% of dams may abort, with abortions occurring in both older and younger animals. In a chronically infected flock, it is often only the first-time mothers that are affected. Infected dams generally abort only once, because they develop immunity.

Treatment: If abortions occur in a flock, it is vital to establish the cause. Affected animals should be removed from the flock, and dead lambs and afterbirths should be disposed of. Your vet can treat animals with tetracylines to prevent epidemic abortion from spreading. This will reduce the duration of an outbreak. A reduction in numbers of cases can be expected after around eight to ten days.

Dams to be served for the first time, and bought-in dams, should be vaccinated before mating (contact your vet). Chlamydial abortion may occur despite **vaccination** because it does not confer 100% protection. Commercial vaccines are available in the UK. It should be used before the mating season.

Chlamydial infection is contagious to **humans**. The main symptoms are a feverish, flu-like disease, an atypical pneumonia and conjunctivitis. Treatment consists of an extended course of tetracyclines. Prompt diagnosis by a doctor is vital. In pregnant women, infection poses a risk of miscarriage.

Campylobacter abortion

General: *Campylobacter* bacteria are spiral-shaped. Infection leads to abortion, usually in the final two weeks of pregnancy. At one time this disease was referred to as vibrionic abortion. The bacteria are ingested orally. They migrate to the uterus via the bloodstream and cause abortion around two weeks later. As a rule, around 20% of pregnant sheep will abort, although the figure is sometimes as high as 50%. Roaming flocks are more rarely affected. Poor paddock hygiene causes bacteria to build up in feed, water and soil. The bacteria can survive here for around 14 to 20 days.

Symptoms: Affected dams are completely **asymptomatic**. The afterbirth is swollen, grey and flaccid.

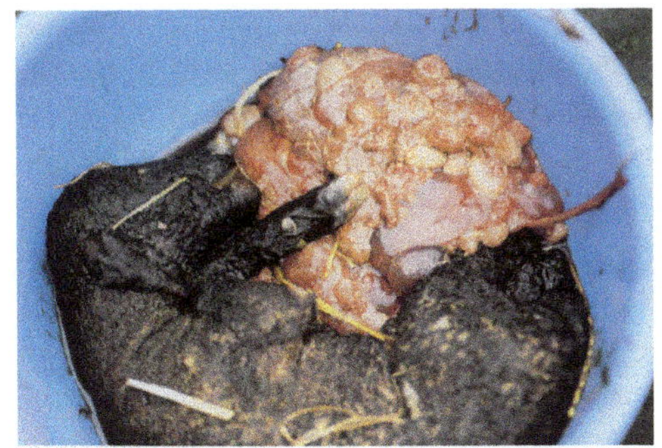

Still-born lamb with slimy, inflamed afterbirth as a result of Chlamydial abortion

Diagnosis: Laboratory testing of foetus and afterbirth, with detection of the characteristic spiral-shaped, highly motile bacteria.

Treatment and preventive measures: To stop bacteria building up, clean and dry conditions and good feed hygiene are vital when keeping pregnant animals. Dams suffering an abortion should be separated from the rest of the flock. Emergency treatment with tetracyclines by your vet is sometimes beneficial.

Other causes of abortion

Salmonella abortion

Main symptoms

- → *Abortions with still births and weakly lambs*

General: The primary cause of this type of abortion is a Salmonella species specific to sheep, *Salmonella abortus ovis.* Animals ingest the bacteria orally. Transmission is via the shedding of bacteria in the urine and dung of infected, asymptomatic animals.

Poor husbandry conditions, lack of feed, feeding errors and bad weather are stressors for the flock and encourage the disease. Around 10% (rarely: 40%) of pregnant infected animals abort in the last third of pregnancy.

Symptoms: Rams and non-pregnant females do not show symptoms of infection but should be regarded as potential chronic shedders. Pregnant dams go through an often unnoticed stage of disease accompanied by fever and sometimes by diarrhoea and vaginal discharge. Abortion occurs two to three weeks after infection, with still births or weakly, infected lambs which die within the first week of life, showing all the signs of salmonellosis.

Diagnosis: Laboratory testing of foetuses and afterbirths is required (bacteriological tests).

Treatment and preventive measures: After a diagnosis of Salmonella abortion, control measures are restricted to antibiotic treatment and hygiene practices. Prevention of salmonellosis by vaccination is only feasible and advisable for certain strains of salmonella. Treatment of still-pregnant dams can be attempted using antibiotics. A suitable approach should be agreed with your vet.

Important measures are thorough **disinfection** of the animals' surroundings and the careful disposal of afterbirths and dead lambs. Salmonella can survive for long periods in the environment (bedding/dung).

When buying in animals, potential chronic shedders should be identified by veterinary faecal testing and then treated. Clean housing and feeding conditions are vital. Stress factors should be minimised during pregnancy. Once a flock has become infected, the ewes usually lamb normally again in the following year.

Brucella abortion

A higher incidence of abortions and weakly lambs can be a sign of brucellosis. Brucellosis is a **notifiable** disease!

Q fever

Sheep and goats become infected via ticks and contact with the agent, which is excreted in massive quantities when infected dams give birth. Abortions tend to be isolated and rarely epidemic. However, humans can also become infected. As in the case of Chlamydial abortion, the agent causes an atypical pneumonia.

Toxoplasmosis

A first-time infection of pregnant animals with *Toxoplasma gondii* can cause abortions. The primary route of infection is ingestion of Toxoplasma from cat faeces.

Disorders of pregnancy

Vaginal prolapse

Main symptoms

- *Straining*
- *Vagina protruding through vulva*

General: Vaginal prolapse is a condition in which the internal tissues of the vagina bulge out through the vulva. It occurs worldwide and in every breed. An inherited predisposition is suspected, so ewes that have had a vaginal prolapse should be excluded from the breeding stock.

Symptoms: Loosening of the vaginal tissues is particularly common in older sheep carrying multiple lambs, due to increasing pressure from the growing uterus. In a multiple pregnancy, the uterus presses not only forwards (on the rumen) but also on the pelvic tissues. This pressure increases further when the animal is lying down, so the prolapse becomes visible. When the animal stands up the prolapse may become smaller or disappear. The prolapsed tissue gets dirty when the affected dam lies down, and can become infected.

Because the urethra is also involved, animals suffer urinary obstruction and an excessive urge to strain. Straining makes the prolapse worse, so it can also be seen when the animal is standing. Excessive straining can lead to a rectal prolapse as well.

Affected sheep arch their backs and grind their teeth. Due to the strong urge to strain, the amniotic membranes can often rupture unnoticed. The birth that this triggers does not progress; the lambs in the uterus can become infected with bacteria and die. In addition, the prolapsed vaginal tissue is very susceptible to injury by other animals.

Treatment: If the prolapse is spotted early, the veterinary surgeon can seal the vagina at the vulva, either by suturing or by using a vulval pin consisting of a metal rod with a wooden ball at each end. If the prolapse is complete (i.e. a large mass of vaginal tissue has prolapsed), the first priority is to check if the foetus is still alive. After cleaning and disinfecting carefully, the veterinary surgeon can then replace the prolapsed tissue and seal the vaginal opening. The ewe should be kept under constant observation to make sure that

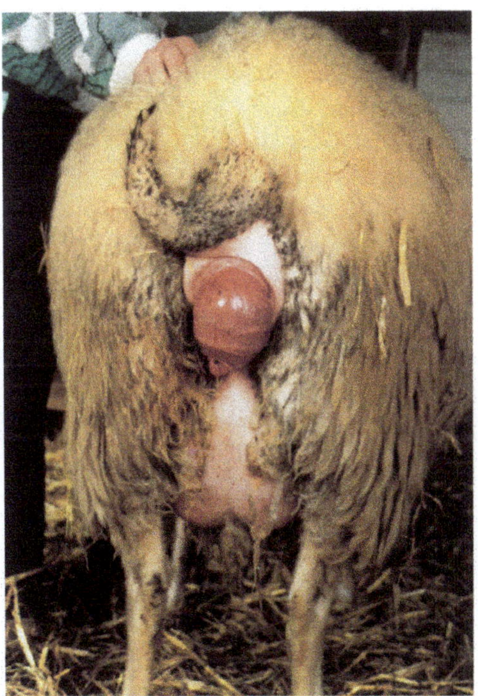

A vaginal prolapse still visible in a standing animal

the start of birth is not missed. The lambing is monitored so that further complications can be tackled quickly.

Uterine torsion

Main symptoms

- ➔ *Restlessness*
- ➔ *Pain*
- ➔ *Straining*
- ➔ *Posture ready for birth*

General: A torsion or twisting of the uterus occurs at the end of pregnancy, before or during birth. In a uterine torsion, the uterus becomes twisted around its own longitudinal axis. **Before birth**, the torsion is located **before** the cervix; **during birth**, the torsion is **in** the cervix.

Uterine torsion has several causes, the main one being vigorous movements by the lambs or sudden leaps or bounds by the dam (overzealous herding by dogs). Turning movements by the foetus may contribute to a uterine torsion. Foetal movements are usually reflex movements caused by external stimuli, e.g. blows or cold water (drunk by the dam). **Symptoms:** A uterine torsion **before birth** is not easy to diagnose because the symptoms are non-specific: restlessness, pain, straining and adopting a posture ready for birth. The body temperature is unchanged but the pulse is raised. Ewes often calm down again, only for the symptoms to reappear after a few hours. Besides being generally restless, affected animals often alternate frequently between lying and standing. A uterine torsion **in the vaginal canal** or cervix, on the other hand, is easier to diagnose. Folds can be felt in the vagina and the cervix is not fully open.

Treatment: A uterine torsion before birth can only be corrected by a veterinary surgeon. The abdominal cavity has to be opened and the twisted uterus properly repositioned. A uterine torsion during birth should also ideally be corrected by a vet due to the high risk of tearing. The uterus needs to be turned in the opposite direction to the torsion, a procedure which can easily result in injury. After reversion, the lambs can be slowly pulled out. The birth canal should be stretched carefully. Once again, there is a high risk of tearing at the torsion site.

Hydrops

Main symptoms

- ➔ *Increase in belly circumference in the last third of pregnancy*
- ➔ *Lumbering gait*

General: Hydrops is the excessive production of amniotic fluid. Fluid can build up in the amnion (inner membrane with mucous-like contents) or the allantois (outer membrane with watery contents). The total content of both membranes is usually around 2.5 to 3 litres. In hydrops it can increase to as much as 12 litres.

The causes of hydrops are not fully understood. Deformities of the lamb and/or dam are thought to play a role.

Symptoms: In the last third of pregnancy, sheep develop a significant increase in belly circumference, a lumbering gait and laboured breathing. Appetite is greatly reduced so affected animals lose weight. Death often follows due to cardiovascular failure.

Diagnosis: Hydrops is not easy to diagnose, as it is often indistinguishable from a multiple pregnancy. However, in hydrops it is rare to be able to feel the foetus. The extreme build-up of fluid is obvious on palpation. If in doubt, always call your vet.

Treatment: Treatment of hydrops depends on its severity and how near the ewe is to lambing. In some situations a caesarean section can save the life of the dam. However, such animals should not be used for further breeding.

All treatment for hydrops involves either surgery or prostaglandin injection and should therefore be carried out by a veterinary surgeon.

Abdominal hernia

Main symptoms

- *Restricted mobility*
- *Distended abdomen*

General: This disease affects older animals (over the age of four) carrying two or more lambs. Due to previous pregnancies, the thin abdominal wall has lost its elasticity. The abdominal muscles tear and the internal organs bulge out underneath the sheep's belly. The pregnant uterus can also extend into the bulge, so that parts of the foetus can be felt below the abdomen.

Symptoms: Depending on the size of the hernia, the sheep's mobility can be severely restricted. Animals often 'go down' and lose their appetite. Affected animals lose weight even though the large belly suggests they are in good nutritional condition. Abdominal hernias can be triggered by sudden movements or trauma such as kicks or blows.

Treatment: Direct surgical intervention is not possible. Treatment should therefore be aimed at preserving the foetus if the lambing due date has not been reached: the dam should be given easily digestible feed, housed on soft deep bedding and monitored closely until lambing. A caesarean section is often required.

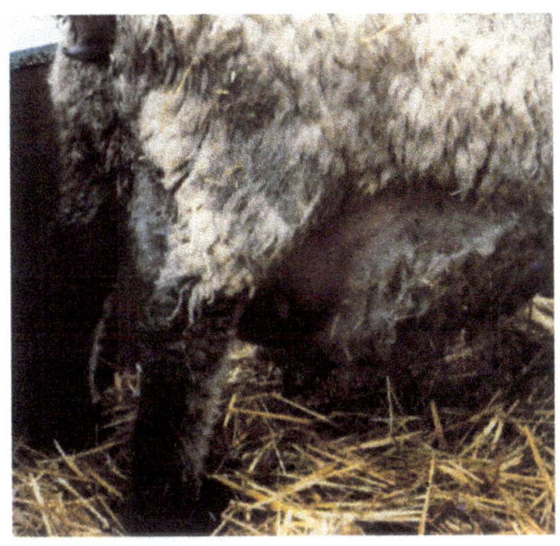

An abdominal hernia in an older sheep

Birth

Normal pregnancy and birth

The **average duration of pregnancy** in sheep and goats is **150 days** (range: 145 to 155 days). By day 30 after fertilisation, a good connection has developed between uterus and foetal membranes. In sheep and goats the birth canal does not usually pose any obstacles to a normal birth.

The approach of birth can be identified by a swollen, bluish-red vulva and 'bagging up' as the udder grows in size in the last third of pregnancy and again a few days before the birth. Immediately before the birth, the teats become firm and point sideways as the milk comes in. Animals spend a lot of time lying down and separate themselves from the flock.

As in other species of animal, birth is divided into three stages, commonly referred to as the three stages of labour:

1. **dilation stage** (passive stage),
2. **expulsion stage** (active stage) and
3. **afterbirth stage**.

The dilation stage does not have any external signs; its function is to open up and soften the cervix and birth canal. This stage ends with the rupture of the water bag. Now begins the actual expulsion of the foetus, accompanied by intense contractions.

The **duration of a normal birth** is up to 30 minutes for singletons and up to 70 minutes for twins. Lambs weigh 4 to 7 kg (singletons) or 3 to 6 kg (twins). In smaller sheep breeds, birth weight is often less than 4 kg.

Once the lambs have been born, the afterbirth stage begins. This should be completed within 3 hours and marks the end of the birth. A normal birth as described above does not require any lambing assistance.

Once the lambs have been born, ewe and lamb start to make contact and develop their relationship by sniffing and licking. Ewes should be allowed plenty of time for this process, as it helps them to recognise their lambs in the flock and encourages a permanent bond.

Preparing for the birth:

The following preparations should be made for lambing time:

1. vaccinate dams promptly for 'pulpy kidney' and tetanus and other clostridial diseases;
2. worm dams;
3. treat dams' hooves in good time (not in the last third of pregnancy);
4. shear the dams' udder and tail regions;
5. set up lambing pens;
6. order milk replacer for sheep, freeze colostrum if possible;
7. get heat lamps ready;
8. order obstetrical lubricant, iodine for disinfecting navels, intrauterine oblets to insert after lambing assistance, intramammary tubes to treat acute mastitis;
9. clean and tidy the lambing shed;
10. order long disposable gloves (to protect yourself against infection).

Birth problems on the part of the dam

Weak contractions

General: Weak contractions occur in older sheep debilitated by chronic illness, abdominal hernia or recumbency. They can also occur in over-fat, inactive animals and in very protracted births.

Symptoms: The expulsion of the foetus by contractions of the uterus and abdominal muscles (abdominal presses) is disrupted. The cervix is open but the foetus has not entered the birth canal.

Treatment: Call your vet, who will attempt to trigger uterine contractions by injecting an oxytocic drug and a calcium solution. With correct positioning of the lamb, the onset of contractions and careful obstetric support, the lamb should now be born. If this does not

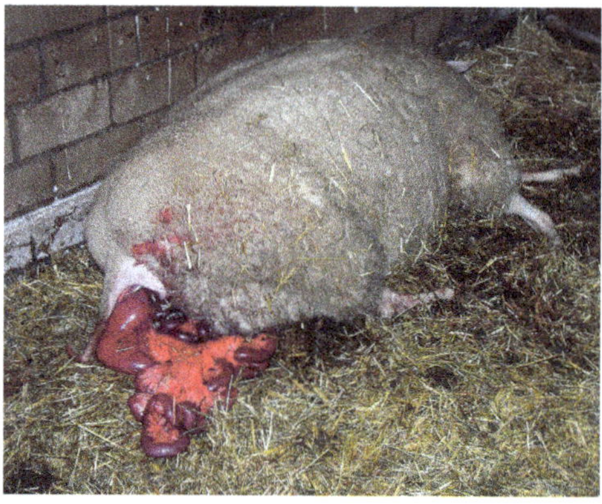

A difficult birth: intestinal prolapse through the vulva after a perforating injury to the cervix. The perforation was identified on post mortem

work either, the vet will perform a caesarean section.

Narrow birth canal ('ringwomb')

Main symptoms

- Birth comes to a halt

General: A narrowing of the birth canal at the cervix, vagina or vulva can prevent lambs from being born despite the presence of contractions.

Symptoms: The dam shows the normal preparations for birth until the contractions begin. The birth then comes to a halt despite continuing contractions. On manual examination, the birth canal is found to be still closed or only partly open.

Treatment: You should be able to gauge how much more assistance you can give without veterinary help. If in any doubt at all, call your vet. You can try to widen a narrow birth canal by massaging carefully. But if your efforts are having no success, never use force to widen the birth canal. You run a high risk of causing injury and bleeding. When assessing your options for lambing assistance, always consider the condition of the dam and the life of the foetus. To obtain live lambs and to save the dam, the veterinary surgeon will sometimes need to perform a caesarean section.

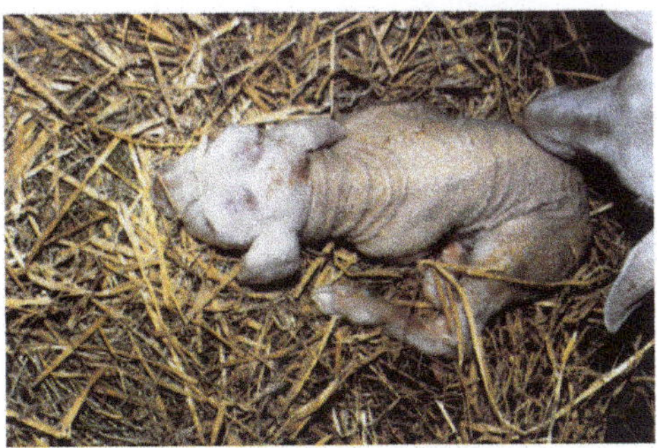

A lamb with a badly swollen head after being stuck in the birth canal for too long. The swelling subsided by itself after a few hours

Birth problems on the part of the lamb

Main symptoms

- Birth comes to a standstill
- Foetus stuck in the birth canal

Position of the foetus

The **normal position** for a lamb about to be born is a forward (anterior) or a backward (posterior) presentation. **Abnormal presentations** are:

- foreleg bent back;
- hindleg bent back;
- head sideways;
- breech.

Oversized foetus

General: The foetus growing in the uterus has become so large that it cannot pass through the birth canal.

Single male lambs invariably grow very large. In addition, particular breed crosses can result in a mismatch between foetus size and width of birth canal.

Deformities such as a bent neck, hydrocephalus, misshapen head or oedema can also affect the lambs' size and prevent them from emerging through the birth canal. An accurate diagnosis is vital, and will allow you to initiate appropriate treatment in consultation with your vet.

Symptoms: The birth begins normally (udder develops, contractions begin, water bag bursts) but there is no sign of the lamb's legs or head. The contractions do not help

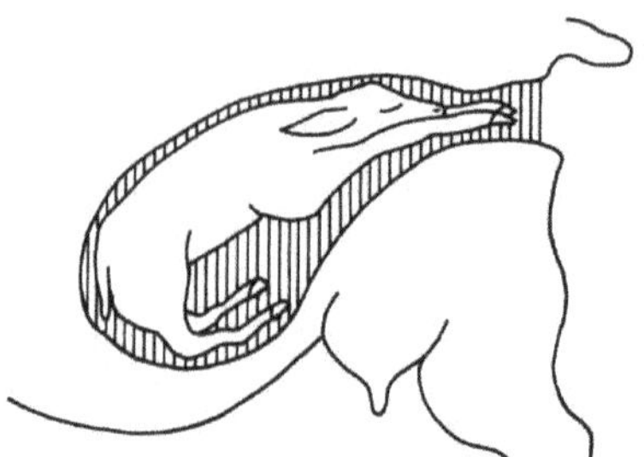

Normal anterior presentation: the front feet appear first, hooves pointing down

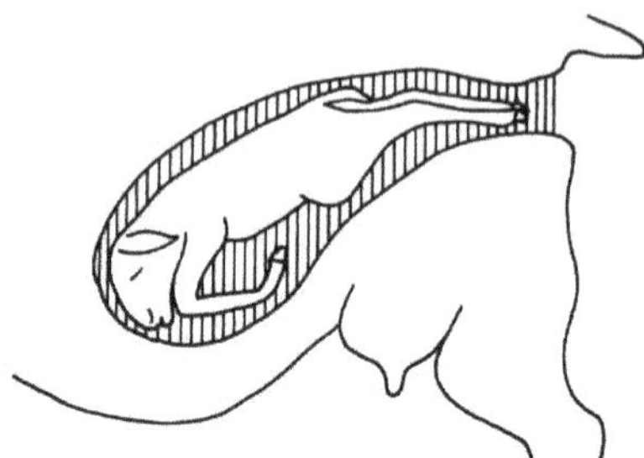

Normal posterior presentation: the hind feet appear first, hooves pointing up

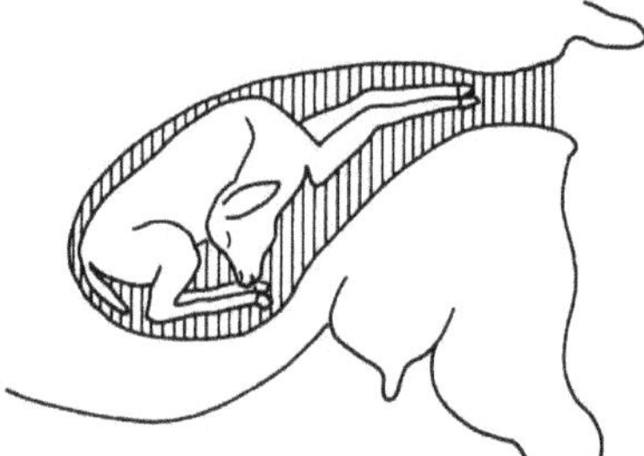

Abnormal anterior presentation with head turned sideways: the lamb cannot be born like this; the head must be brought forward

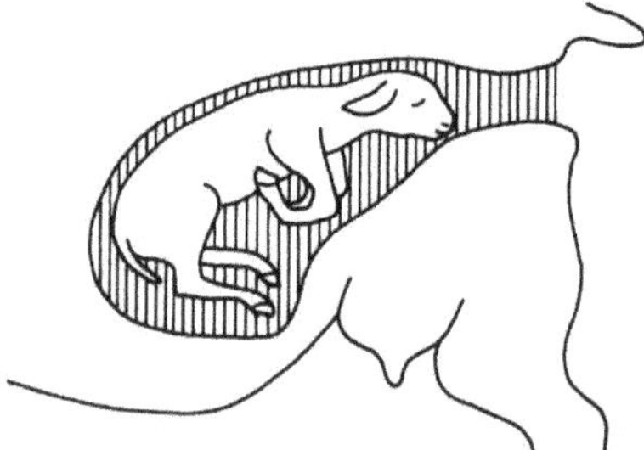

Abnormal anterior presentation with retained forelimbs: the forelimbs must be brought forward for the lamb to be born

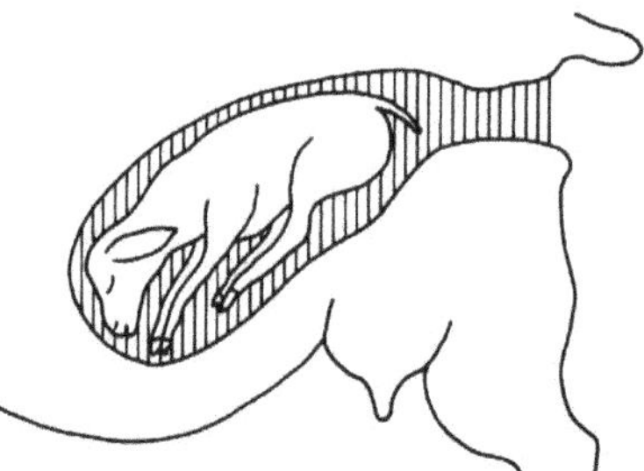

Abnormal posterior presentation with hindlimbs under the body: for the lamb to be born, it needs to be adjusted to a normal posterior presentation

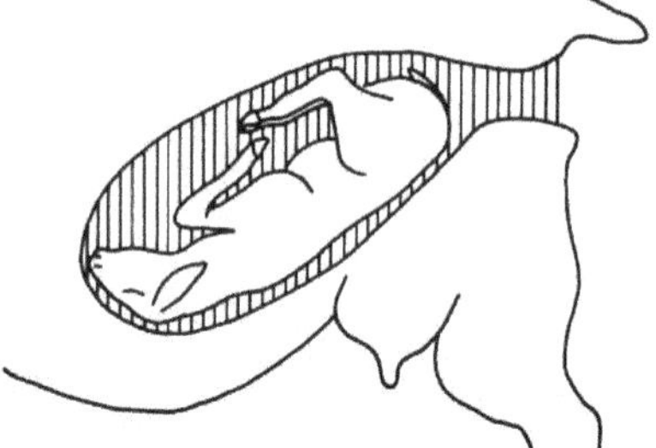

Abnormal upside-down posterior presentation with hindlimbs under the body: the lamb needs to be adjusted to a normal presentation before it can be born

Normal and abnormal presentations of the lamb during birth

the birth to progress but simply exhaust the mother. On examination, a foetus can be felt in the birth canal. The foetus is very large, indicating a mismatch between foetus size and the width of the birth canal. In this case the veterinary surgeon will perform a caesarean section to save both mother and lamb.

Twins in the birth canal

General: Two foetuses entering the birth canal at the same time leads to the lambs becoming wedged and brings the birth to a standstill.

Symptoms: All of the signs point towards a normal birth but then no lamb appears. On manual examination, multiple limbs, heads or rumps can be felt inside the pelvis. It is usually very difficult to tell which body part belongs to which lamb.

Treatment: Elevate the dam's pelvis and carefully push the lambs back in. Tie a rope round the legs of the lamb furthest forward in the birth canal and pull gently while pushing the other lamb back into the uterus. Rotate the first lamb into normal position and pull it out very carefully.

Note: Use plenty of lubricant!

Lambing assistance

Lambing assistance should be given only in the following cases:

1. the water bag has burst and no lamb has appeared after an hour;
2. the birth comes to a standstill;
3. the lamb becomes stuck in the birth canal.

Important **precautions** before giving lambing assistance:

1. Cleanliness:

   - clean the ewe's anus and vulva with soap solution and then with disinfectant;
   - move the ewe onto fresh bedding;
   - wash your hands, forearms and upper arms; keep fingernails short and clean.

2. Use plenty of lubricant when examining the birth canal.
3. All interventions should be carried out carefully and without using force or violence. It is extremely easy to tear the uterus and injure the birth canal.
4. Time your pulling to coincide with the mother's contractions.
5. If no progress is being made, call your vet.

If there are specific problems on the part of dam or lamb, the following assistance can be given:

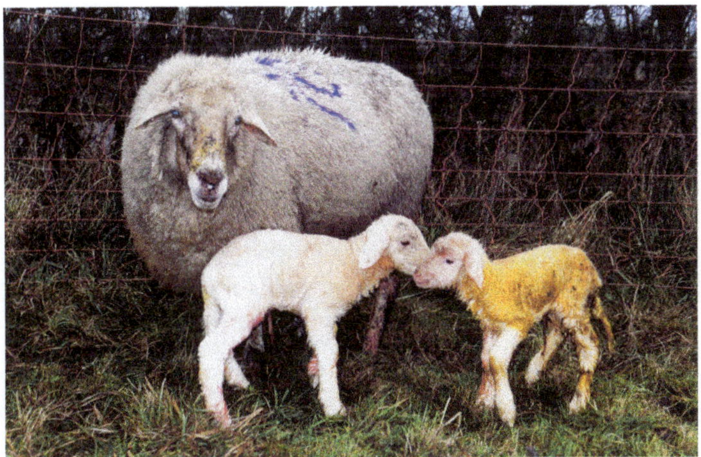

Ewe with healthy twins soon after birth

- **Weak contractions:** check the lamb's position and how open the birth canal is, inject an oxytocic drug (vet), pull the lamb out carefully.
- **Narrow birth canal** (cervix): use two fingers to open the cervix; use lubricant! If there is no progress after 15 minutes, call your vet.
- **Oversized lamb:**
  - **Head stuck:** push the head back carefully, apply lubricant, pull the lamb out carefully by the head, with outside assistance.
  - **Shoulders stuck:** pull carefully on the forelegs, alternating between legs; use lubricant!
  - **Pelvis stuck:** pull carefully on the forelegs, rotating the body; use lubricant!
- **Malpositions:** Two lambs in the birth canal: push one lamb back into the uterus, apply lubricant, rotate into normal birth position, tie obstetric ropes to legs, use lubricant, pull out carefully. In multiple births, push lambs back into the uterus, check ownership of heads and legs, rotate into normal birth position, use lubricant, pull out carefully.

Injuries to the birth canal

Main symptoms

- *Bleeding from vulva*

General: Injuries can occur in the uterus, cervix and vagina.

Injuries to the cervix occur due to a lack of care during manual interventions, extraction of large lambs, or if the cervix was not open enough. If the foetus is malpositioned, the uterus can be punctured or injured during strong contractions.

Injuries to the vagina generally occur after protracted births accompanied by swelling or drying of the birth canal and incorrect, forceful extraction of lambs.

Symptoms: Injuries to the uterus, cervix and vagina can cause bleeding. Bleeding in the uterus stays within the uterine cavity at first and is not immediately visible. If the bleeding is in the cervix or vagina, blood will be seen coming from the vulva. The amount of blood depends on how severe the injury is. If the wall of the uterus has been punctured, bleeding is into the abdominal cavity and is not visible from the outside. Ewes become weak and, depending on the extent of the injury, develop pale mucous membranes. Because a bacterial infection is usually present as well, they have a high temperature.

Treatment: Minor, superficial injuries generally heal without complications. More extensive injuries should be seen by your vet and treated with medication to stem the bleeding. Complications are likely at the next lambing. If the uterus is punctured, the only option for the ewe is emergency euthanasia.

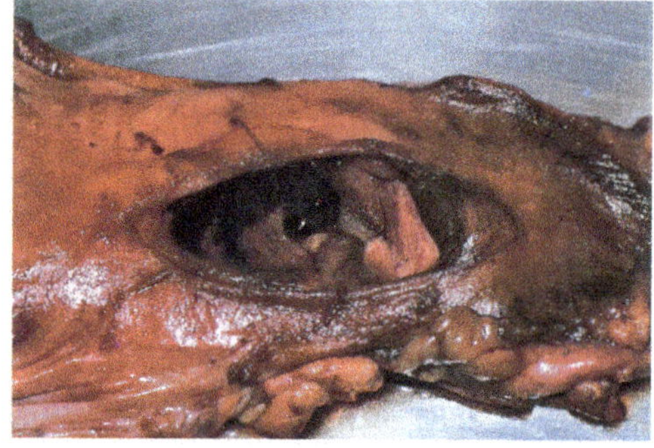

Punctured uterus due to incorrect lambing assistance. The injury was detected after the death of the ewe

Note: All lambing assistance should be carried out carefully, gently and without using force. Use plenty of lubricant! Put an antibiotic pessary into the uterus after giving lambing assistance.

Diseases after the birth

Uterine prolapse

Main symptoms

- → *Part of the uterus appears at the vulva*

General: A prolapsed or everted uterus can occur after a difficult birth, but sometimes even after a normal birth. It often follows weak contractions or a twin birth. Overfeeding during pregnancy increases the rate of uterine prolapse in a flock.

Symptoms: Sheep and goats neglect their lambs, show signs of straining and arch their backs. Parts of the uterus appear at the vulva. If the prolapse occurred some time ago, the uterus may be reddish-blue and dirtied with straw, dung and earth.

Treatment: Proper treatment should be left to your vet, especially as prolapses can recur soon after being replaced.

To replace a prolapse, the animal's pelvis must be elevated. The prolapsed tissue is thoroughly cleaned and disinfected with a warm disinfectant soap solution, and then coated with lubricant. The prolapse can be replaced by pushing gently with the flat of both hands. To avoid a recurrence, the vet should suture the vulva closed.

Preventive measures: Uterine prolapse cannot always be prevented. Correct feeding during pregnancy is important but weak contractions and slack ligaments in the mother play a role and are difficult to foresee. Sheep and goats that have had a uterine prolapse should be culled from the breeding stock.

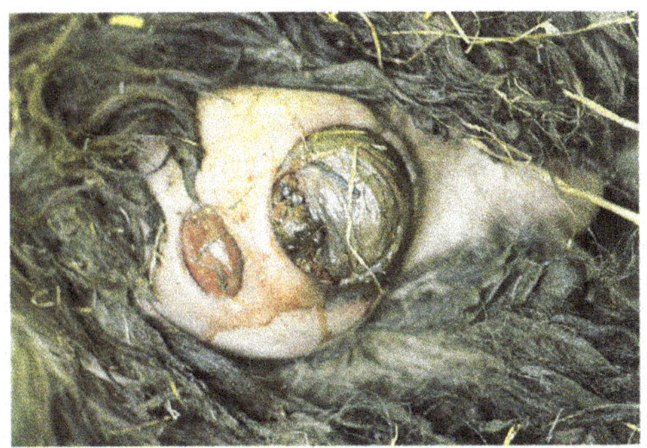

Right: uterine prolapse

Metritis

Main symptoms

- → *Discharge from vulva*
- → *Fever*
- → *Lethargy*

General: Metritis is an infection of the uterus following a protracted or disrupted delivery, inexpert lambing assistance or incomplete expulsion of the afterbirth. It often results in a severe impairment of the animal's overall condition. The first symptoms usually go unnoticed, which allows various species of bacteria to multiply undisturbed and spread throughout the body.

Symptoms: Dams are lethargic and go off their food. They develop a high temperature (40°C to 41°C), tight abdomen and pale, bluish mucous membranes. Due to lack of milk, lambs are undernourished and their development is retarded. A foul-smelling reddish-brown discharge comes from the vulva. In sheep, the wool can fall out in large clumps.

Treatment: In addition to multiple treatments with antibiotics and drugs to protect the liver, the vet will remove any pieces of retained afterbirth. Veterinary care should continue until the dam's fever subsides and her general condition improves.

Retained afterbirth

General: A retained afterbirth is rare following a normal delivery. The dam should pass the afterbirth within 12 hours after the birth.

Premature births, multiple births or a lack of calcium and/or magnesium can trigger retention of the afterbirth.

Symptoms: The passing of the afterbirth is not normally monitored in sheep or goats because complications are rare. The signs of a retained afterbirth are vaginal discharge and tissue trailing from the vulva. In advanced cases, sheep show general ill health (fever, lethargy) and refuse to eat.

Treatment: Pull carefully when removing a retained placenta, as tugging strongly will cause the animal to strain, which could trigger a uterine prolapse. The vet will insert a uterine pessary and treat the animal with antibiotics. Treatment should continue until the animal has recovered.

Oblets and antibiotics should also be used if active assistance has been given during the birth, as interventions in the birth canal can introduce bacteria into the uterus.

Newborn lambs

Care and nutrition

After a natural birth, the mother/lamb relationship is forged immediately by licking, grooming and sniffing.

If birth takes place with outside assistance, mother and lamb must be given the opportunity to make contact, i.e. lambs should be taken to the mother immediately.

Lambs attempt to get up soon after birth; they should be able to stand on their own within 30 minutes. If lambs have been weakened by the birth, attempts to stand can lead to exhaustion and the mother will lose interest in the weakly lamb. Mothers usually abandon exhausted lambs.

Proper **navel disinfection** should be practised to avoid infection. The best treatment is tincture of iodine. Dip the fresh navel in a container of iodine, or pull the navel cord apart slightly and drip some iodine in. Treating the navel with an antibiotic spray is easy and convenient but does not disinfect or dry the navel cord sufficiently, leading to infection and losses of lambs.

The **meconium**, which plugs the lamb's intestines up until birth, normally passes easily within a day. If meconium is retained, an enema can be attempted using clean, lukewarm water. Adding 20 ml of liquid paraffin improves lubrication. Support the process by massaging the lamb's abdomen.

Drinking **colostrum** as early as possible is essential for newborn lambs. The first milk

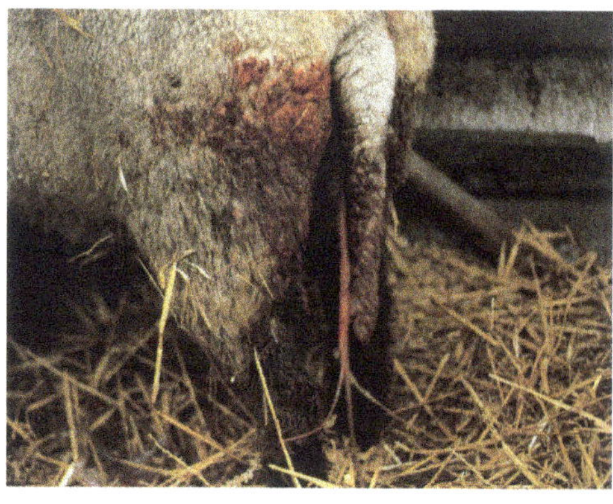

Trailing afterbirth membranes still to be passed after a recent birth

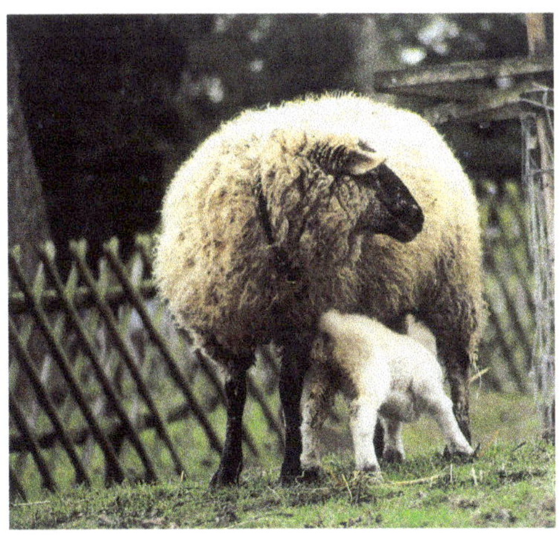

A healthy mother/lamb relationship

contains antibodies against infection and supplies the lamb with energy. The lamb should drink around 100 ml of colostrum within the first 24 hours. After this the lamb can no longer fully utilise the antibody-rich milk because the absorption of antibodies from the gut falls off sharply after 24 hours. In the gut itself, however, the mother's milk continues to protect the lambs against diarrhoeal diseases. This is why weak or abandoned lambs should be fed with colostrum artificially. Give them multiple small portions (20 to 30 ml) of either frozen colostrum or milk from a dam that lambed at the same time as their own mother. Frozen colostrum can be kept for around nine months.

Mothers that have given birth to dead lambs can be used to foster other lambs. To encourage acceptance, smear foster lambs with birth mucus from the dead lamb, or rub them with its fleece. Despite these steps, dams will not always accept a strange lamb. Another way to encourage fostering is to put lamb and dam together in a shared pen. Tie the dam to the bars in such a way that the lamb can suckle without being driven off by defensive movements or kicks from the dam. Repeat this procedure several times a day. After four to five days, it often succeeds in getting dam and lamb accustomed to each other.

If lambs are to be reared without their mothers, you will need to use a **milk replacer**. In the first few days, check that the lambs are getting used to the drinkers. If lambs are being bottle-reared, a three-hourly feeding rhythm should be maintained in the first few days, with the volume of milk being gradually increased.

Bottle-reared lambs quickly become used to humans and rarely lose this familiarity as adult sheep. They approach people and are very trusting. This is not always an advantage.

Diseases

Breathing difficulties

General: Levels of oxygen in the lamb's blood fall during birth, so breathing must start immediately after birth in order to make up the deficiency.

Symptoms: Lambs breathe weakly or not at all. The mucous membranes are bluish and the head is outstretched.

Treatment: Clear the nostrils of any fluids from the birth. In some cases, mucus may have to be removed with a syringe or a tube. Pouring cold water on to the torso and massaging carefully encourages breathing. Swinging the lamb with its head down should be attempted only very carefully, while supporting the head and neck, to avoid injury to the neck vertebrae. Breathing stimulants applied in drops on to the tongue can help the lamb to breathe spontaneously.

Lack of milk (lack of energy)

General: Lambs must receive colostrum within the first 24 hours of life. Besides antibodies, colostrum contains readily available energy resources that the lamb's metabolism needs in order to stabilise its body temperature. A lack of milk leads to a life-threatening drop in body temperature.

Symptoms: Lambs shiver and arch their backs. Their movements become uncontrolled. If untreated, this leads to downer animals and death.

Treatment: Rub the lambs dry, put them under a heat lamp and give them some milk. Injecting dextrose solution under the skin can be helpful (5% solution, 10 to 15 ml at various sites).

Navel ill

General: If navels are not properly disinfected soon after birth, bacteria can enter the navel cord and cause localised or generalised infections.

Symptoms: In a local infection, a pus-filled abscess develops at the navel. From here, bacteria can migrate to the liver and cause abscesses there as well. Bacteria can also cause arthritis. Joints become swollen, painful and hot to the touch. Lambs develop a fever, stop suckling and become weak. Death follows within a few days.

Treatment: If infection is spotted early, affected lambs can be saved by repeated doses of antibiotics. In cases of advanced arthritis, treatment is pointless.

Preventive measures: With thorough navel disinfection colostrum feeding, clean lambing areas with fresh bedding and adequate birth monitoring, navel ill is almost entirely preventable.

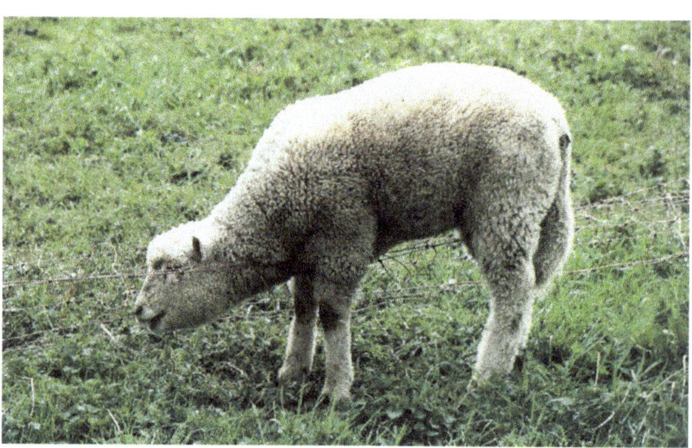

A lamb caught up in the fence

22

Diseases particularly affecting goats

Infectious diseases

Almost all infectious diseases of sheep also occur in goats. The following section describes a number of diseases that are seen more often in goats.

Caprine arthritis-encephalitis (CAE)

Main symptoms: Brain form

- → *Ataxia*
- → *Stiff gait*
- → *Balance problems*

Main symptoms: Joint form

- → *Swollen joints*
- → *Lameness*
- → *Rough coat*

General: Caprine arthritis-encephalitis (CAE) is a chronic, progressive viral infection affecting goats. It is the most important infectious disease of goats and all breeding associations should control it by means of a voluntary programme. The virus is related to but distinct from maedi-visna virus in sheep. It is transmitted to kids in the colostrum of virus-positive does, and directly from animal to animal via close contact.

Symptoms: Two forms of the disease are distinguished:

1. **Brain form**: This mainly affects kids between two and four months old, more rarely adult animals. Locomotor disorders such as an unsteady gait, ataxia and paralysis are observed. Balance problems are common. Signs of pneumonia may also be seen.
2. **Joint form:** Adult animals lose weight and develop a rough, shaggy coat. The carpal joints become swollen. This swelling leads to increasing lameness, until the animals can only walk on their knees. In females, the swollen joints are accompanied by a drop in milk yield.

Diagnosis: The typical symptoms of this disease are confirmed by a laboratory blood test to detect the specific antibodies.

Treatment: There is no specific treatment. Good husbandry conditions and optimum nutrition can promote recovery.

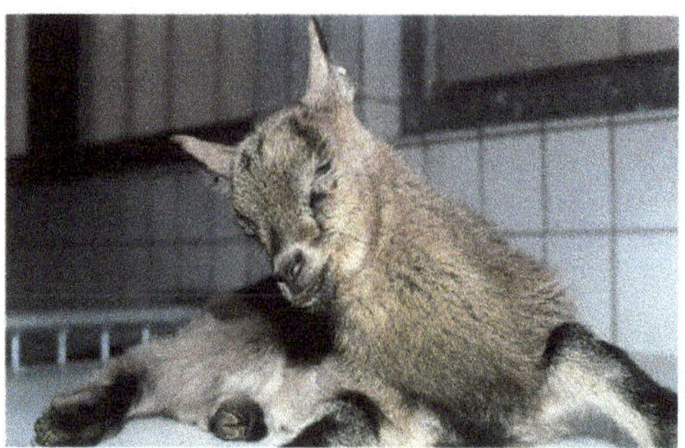

This kid has serious problems with its balance and movement

Preventive measures: The aim of any **control programme** should be to create herds that are free of CAE. This sort of programme is similar to maedi-visna control in sheep:

1. Blood testing of all animals over six months old.
2. A herd is declared disease free if all animals test negative in three successive blood tests conducted 6 to 12 months apart.
3. The herd remains disease free if all animals are tested annually with negative results.
4. A herd loses its disease-free status:
   - if it does not remain a closed population;
   - if it buys in positive or untested animals.
5. The disease can be eradicated in infected herds by:
   - culling all CAE-positive animals, including offspring in the case of females;
   - separate housing and limited use of CAE-positive animals;
   - motherless rearing of kids born to CAE-positive mothers.

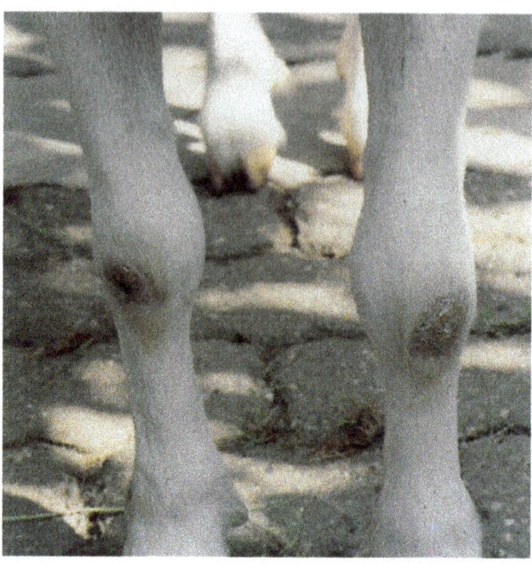

Swollen knee joints in a case of CAE

As a basic principle, eradication programmes such as these specify that only animals from CAE-free herds can be taken to events such as auctions or performance tests.

Because eradication programmes are not currently funded and CAE is not notifiable, eradication is implemented by the regional associations on a voluntary basis. To create CAE-free herds which can serve as a foundation for further breeding, as many breeders as possible should participate. Eradication programmes of this type have been carried out successfully in Switzerland and Austria.

Metabolic disorders

Copper toxicity (enzootic ataxia) and cerebrocortical necrosis

Main symptoms: Copper deficiency

- *Acute: diarrhoea, haematuria, convulsions, anaemia*
- *Chronic: weight loss, jaundice, haematuria, eczema*

Main symptoms: Cerebrocortical necrosis

- → *Movement disorders*
- → *Animals lying on sides with heads stretched out*
- → *Convulsions*

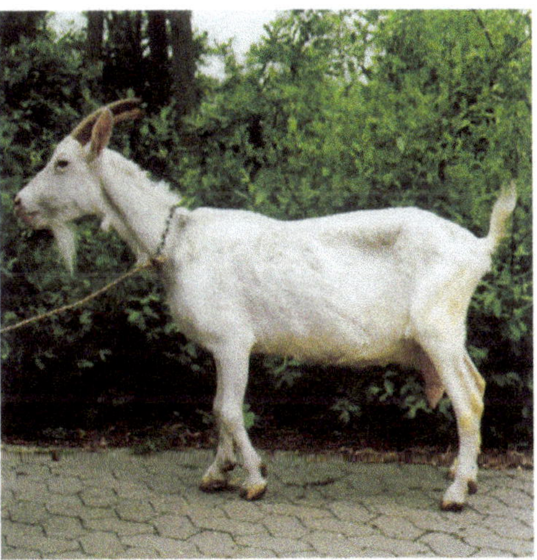

Emaciation and arthritis are typical symptoms of CAE

General: A deficiency of copper in the first few weeks of life results in developmental disorders of the nervous system in kids, and a lack of vitamin B leads to a disease of the central nervous system with symptoms which start to appear as brain cells die (necrosis).

Iodine deficiency

Main symptoms

- → *Enlargement of the thyroid gland*
- → *Goitre*

General: In certain regions such as the Alps, an iodine deficiency in fodder plants leads to a lack of iodine in the diet and the development of a goitre in adult animals and newborn kids.

A distinction is drawn between primary iodine deficiency, due to a lack of iodine in the diet, and secondary iodine deficiency, caused by eating certain plants containing substances which promote thyroid growth and lock up the iodine in the food.

Symptoms: Kids are stillborn or weak. Live-born kids die soon after birth due to suffocation. A clear enlargement of the thyroid gland can be seen. Adult animals also show enlarged thyroid glands but are otherwise free of symptoms.

Treatment and preventive measures: An acute iodine deficiency can be treated by giving tincture of iodine (0.2 ml per day for 14 days). Treatment should not be continued for any longer due to the risk of iodine poisoning. In iodine-deficient regions, iodine can be added to the mineral feed (0.01%). Iodine treatment is generally too late in weak newborn kids with goitre.

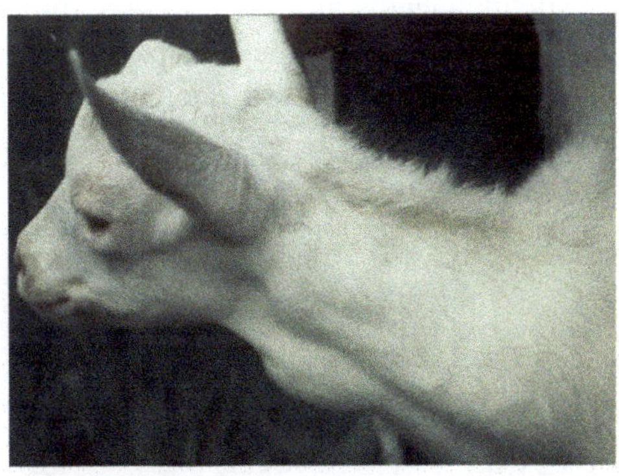

Kid with an iodine deficiency goitre

Skin and coat

Demodectic mites (hair follicle mites, demodectic mange)

Main symptoms

- *Hair loss*
- *Crusts and pustules*
- *No itching*

General: Demodectic mange is an infection of the hair follicles caused by a species of mite which occurs in animals worldwide, including goats. It is less common in sheep.

Symptoms: This mite infection is transmitted by animal-to-animal contact and causes hair loss, crusting and pustules. The pustules are filled with a thick, dry secretion. When the contents are expressed, large numbers of mites can be detected under the microscope. Unlike other forms of mange, demodectic mange does not cause itching. Demodex mites can also be detected in apparently healthy animals; the symptoms described above tend to be seen in older animals weakened by disease or poor husbandry and feeding conditions.

Treatment and preventive measures: Good husbandry and feeding causes the symptoms to disappear: however, this does not mean that the mites have been eliminated.

Baths, dips or sprays containing chemicals to control external parasites help to limit the disease. Treatment with macrocyclic lactones can be given under veterinary supervision.

Ringworm (trichophytia)

Main symptoms

- *Flaky, crusted areas of skin, usually on the head*

General: This fungal skin disease occurs worldwide in all animals and also in humans. It is occasionally observed in goats, without causing significant economic losses. However, goats can be a source of infection for humans.

Infection: The fungus is transmitted by animal-to-animal contact; dogs can also be vectors. Contaminated equipment such as feeders, vehicles and fences can also spread the disease.

Symptoms: Affected animals show raw, flaky or crusted patches of skin on the head, legs and tail root. The severe itching leads to chafing or rubbing and bloody crusts can develop.

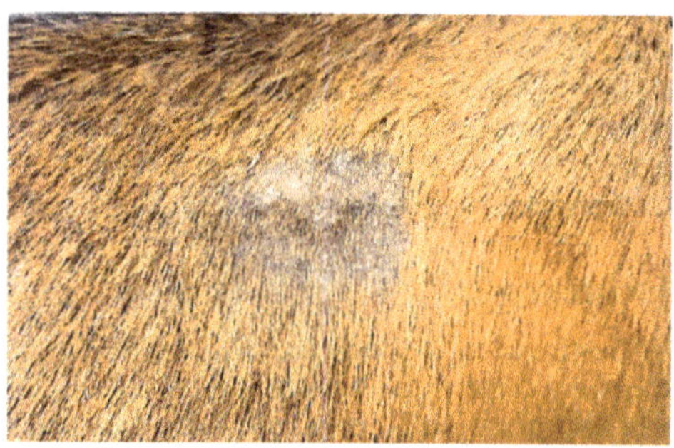

Demodex mites cause hair loss and pustules

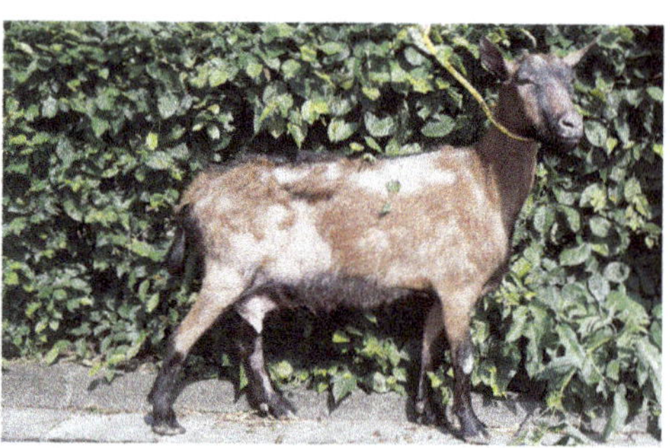

A goat with ringworm

Treatment: The disease often resolves by itself if housing and feeding conditions are improved. The skin lesions can be treated with topical antimycotic (antifungal) agents. Treatment should continue for some time after a visible improvement has occurred.

Note: Humans can catch the infection!

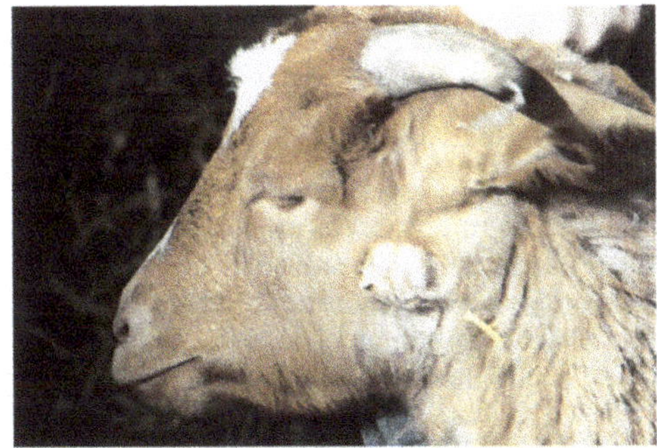

Thick pus forms in infected lymph nodes in the head. This animal is relatively unaffected by the disease

Caseous lymphadenitis (CLA; pseudotuberculosis) of sheep and goats

Main symptoms

- *Caseous inflammation of skin lymph nodes*
- *Thick, greenish pus*

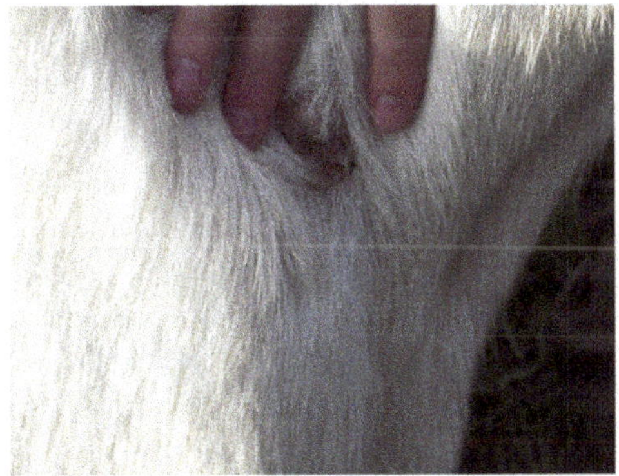

Pseudotuberculosis abscess on a goat's neck

General: Caseous lymphadenitis is a chronic contagious disease of the skin lymph nodes and skin lymph vessels. Lymph nodes of internal organs can also be affected. The agent responsible is the bacterium *Corynebacterium pseudotuberculosis.*

Symptoms: The pus from erupting skin abscesses contains large numbers of bacteria that spread the infection through close contact with other animals, mainly via minor skin wounds. Such wounds tend to occur on the head in goats, which often injure themselves while browsing on thorny shrubs and bushes.

Horned goats often sustain head injuries during battles over pecking order. In caseous lymphadenitis the lymph vessels become inflamed and contain a caseous (cheese-like) material. String-like swellings with open abscesses develop. A thick, greenish pus drains from these abscesses. Goats with the disease often appear relatively unaffected. In a serious episode, however, animals become emaciated and sometimes develop breathing difficulties.

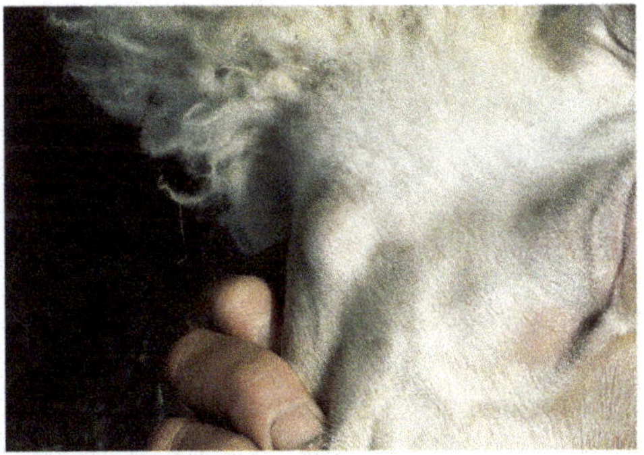

Pseudotuberculosis abscess on a sheep's lower jaw.

The disease is often spread by buying in animals with an undetected infection.

Treatment and preventive measures: If skin lesions are in the initial stages, antibiotic treatment can be attempted. However, euthanasia is recommended if extensive areas of skin are affected and there are obvious breathing difficulties. Risks of injury can be reduced by improving the conditions in which animals are kept. Consistent vaccination with a herd-specific vaccine can also help to eliminate the disease in an affected herd.

Diseases of the digestive organs

Intestinal parasites

For goat keepers, it is important to know that parasites can be transmitted between sheep and goats, and that goats infested with gastrointestinal worms can go a long time without showing clear symptoms, only to become lethargic, go off their food and suffer an apparently 'sudden' death.

Many sheep wormers do not have the same efficacy in goats. In some cases the dose will need to be increased. Ask your vet or your local animal health service. Often, however, you will have to use wormers that are not licensed for goats.

Because these products are generally licensed for sheep, your vet will be able to authorise 'off-label use'.

Johne's disease (paratuberculosis)

General: This disease can also occur in goats. The agents are excreted into the environment and become dispersed.

Diseases of dairy goats

Calcium and magnesium deficiency

Main symptoms: Calcium deficiency in late pregnancy

- *Movement disorders*
- *'Downer' animals with outstretched necks*

Main symptoms: Magnesium deficiency

- *'Downer' animals*
- *Convulsions*
- *Excessive salivation*

General: In goats, as in sheep, calcium deficiency manifests as a disturbance of calcium metabolism affecting older goats in late pregnancy. In the final stages of pregnancy the demand for calcium increases as it is used to build bone in the foetus. The dam needs to supply the growing kid with calcium.

Magnesium deficiency (**grass tetany**) usually occurs after turning goats out onto fast-growing grass pasture. Animals go down and show convulsion-like symptoms.

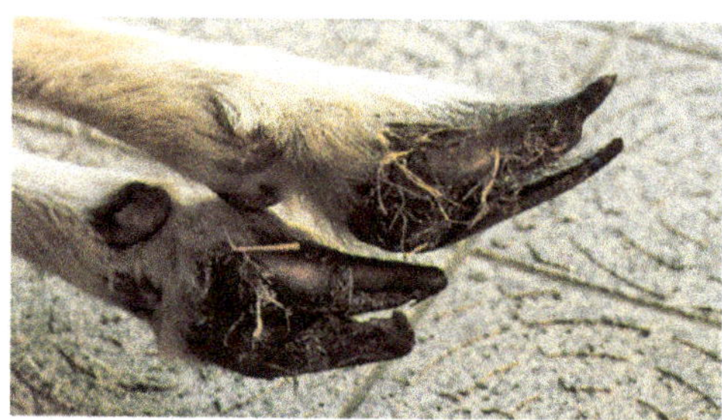

Hoof care: poor hoof care affects goats as well as sheep

Pregnancy toxaemia (ketosis)

Main symptoms

- → *Lethargy*
- → *Reduced rumen activity*
- → *'Downer' animals*
- → *Rapid breathing*

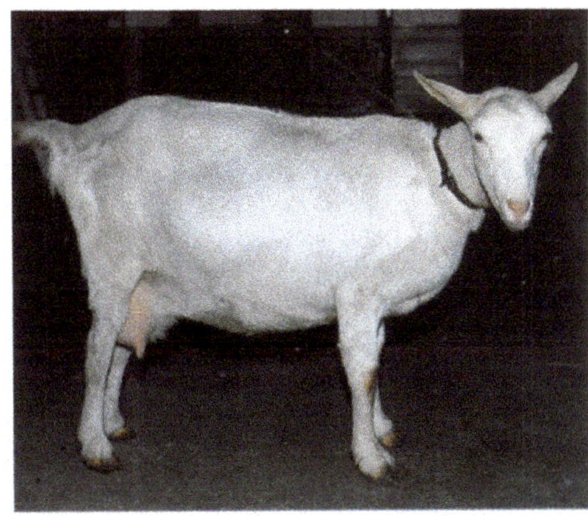

Heavily pregnant doe with ataxic gait. The animal was treated successfully and delivered healthy kids

General: Goats in late pregnancy (usually carrying multiple kids) sometimes develop an acute metabolic disorder accompanied by a fall in blood sugar levels.

Symptoms: In the early stages of the disease, animals become lethargic and go off their food. Rumen activity stops or becomes sluggish. In the acute stages, animals go down. Their mucous membranes look dirty or pale and their breathing is rapid. Their breath smells fruity. Blood tests indicate reduced blood sugar levels. Urine testing shows a rise in ketone bodies.

Treatment: To raise blood sugar levels in affected animals, the vet will give an injection of glucose into the vein.

23

Supplement on viral diseases

Bluetongue disease (BT)

Main symptoms

- ➔ *Fever (40°C), lameness*
- ➔ *Reddening and swelling of mucosae of lips and mouth, muzzle, eyelids*
- ➔ *Reddened, swollen scrotum or udder skin*

General: Bluetongue is an infectious disease of domestic and wild ruminants caused by a virus (orbivirus) and transmitted by midges of the genus *Culicoides*. This disease was identified north of the Alps for the first time in August 2006, with virus serotype 8. The disease spread quickly throughout Germany and other European countries, in some cases causing dramatic losses among sheep and cattle.

The virus (orbivirus) is transmitted by various native species of the blood-sucking Culicoides midge, which can be dispersed over wide areas by the wind. The midges have a variety of breeding sites, including stagnant water, puddles, hollow trees, rotting leaves, dung heaps and slurry pits, so targeted control is virtually impossible.

Symptoms: The first symptoms appear 4 to 12 days after an animal has been bitten by an infected midge. They include fever (up to 40°C), fatigue, lameness and a drooping head. These are followed by reddening and swelling of the mucosae of the lips and mouth, and swelling of the muzzle and eyelids. The hooves become reddened and inflamed above the coronary band. In rams, the scrotum is red and inflamed; in ewes, the skin of the udder is affected. The midge bites are easy to see. A blue discolouration of the tongue has been observed in a few cases. On post mortem, bleeding and ulcers are found in the tongue, mouth, rumen lining and heart muscle.

Diagnosis: Infection is confirmed in the laboratory by means of serology and PCR tests.

Differential diagnosis: Foot-and-mouth disease, Border disease, sheep pox, Orf, photosensitivity.

Treatment and control: Bluetongue is a **notifiable** disease, which means that all control measures are initiated by the competent veterinary office. Treatment with antibiotics and anti-inflammatories helps to alleviate the disease but deaths will nevertheless occur. Midge repellents are of variable efficacy in preventing infection.

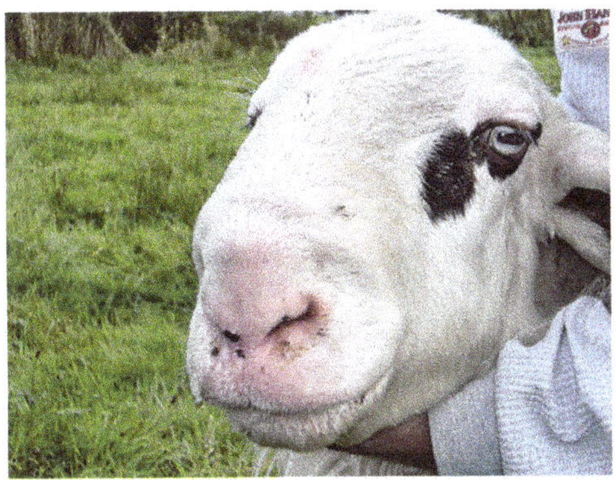

Acute bluetongue: swollen head

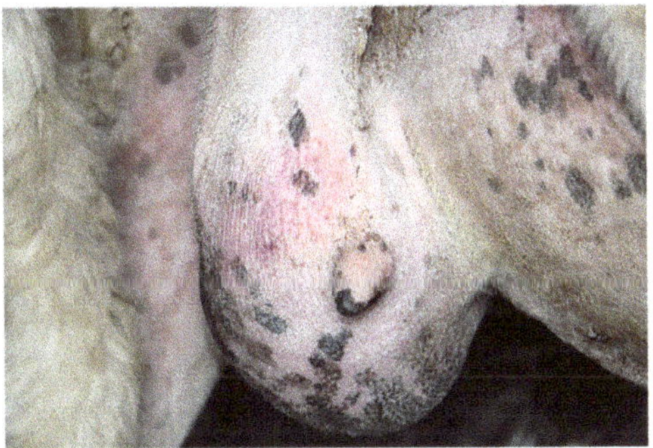

Acute bluetongue: reddening around midge bites on the udder

Prevention: Preventive vaccination is the only reliable method of protection. Sheep and goats should be vaccinated once per animal in accordance with veterinary advice.

Schmallenberg virus infection

Main symptoms

- → *Malformations of the spine, limbs, lower jaw, twisted neck*
- → *Difficult births*

General: In December 2011 an increased incidence of malformations was observed in lambs. Similar defects were noticed in kids a month later. The virus was first detected in sheep in January 2012. The new virus was called 'Schmallenberg virus' (SBV) after the place where it was initially detected. It belongs to the Akabane complex viruses and is a new orthobunyavirus. Calves are also affected, resulting in malformations and still births. Schmallenberg virus infection was demonstrated in many European countries in 2012, including NL, B, LUX, F and UK.

Infection: The virus is transmitted by native species of the blood-sucking Culicoides midge. If dams are bitten by infected midges at a particular stage of pregnancy, the virus settles in the uterus and causes defects in the unborn lamb. The sensitive time window for infection (when some defects are very severe) is thought to be from days 28 to 56 of pregnancy. Before 28 days, the foetus is reabsorbed. If infection occurs after 56 days, lambs are usually born healthy.

Symptoms: Still-born and live-born lambs show serious defects such as bent limbs and spines, twisted neck (torticollis), and a short lower jaw (brachygnathia). Post mortem reveals brain malformations such as hydrocephalus and cerebellar hypoplasia. Depending on the severity of the defects,

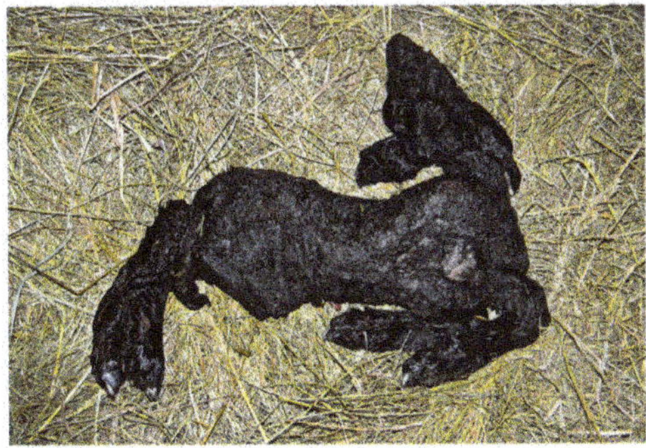

Schmallenberg virus infection: torticollis in a newborn lamb

surviving lambs are non-viable or need to be euthanased.

Unlike dairy cows, adult ewes show no symptoms after infection. At birth, however, the defects can cause difficulties requiring a caesarian section or euthanasia of the dam. Sheep farmers report poor fertility and returns to oestrus during the midge season. In a twin birth, often one lamb is healthy while the other is deformed.

Diagnosis: On post mortem of deformed lambs, the virus can be isolated from brain material. It can often be detected in the meconium as well. Serological testing will clarify the situation for the rest of the flock. Deformed lambs should therefore be tested as a matter of urgency.

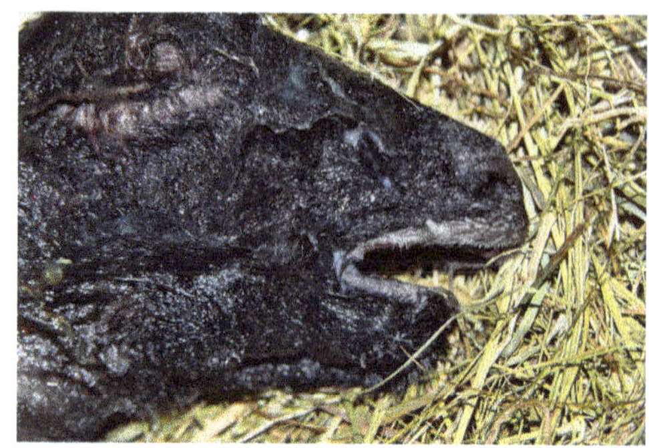

Schmallenberg virus infection: brachygnathia in a newborn lamb

Treatment and control: A vaccine is already licensed in the UK (summer 2013). Midge repellents can limit infection but not prevent it entirely.

Resources

Glossary

Anthelmintics Wormers; products which control internal parasites.

Antibiotics Medicines which kill or inhibit the growth of micro-organisms (bacteria).

Antibodies Naturally occurring proteins in the body which protect against infection.

Antimycotics Medicines that kill or inhibit the growth of fungal organisms.

Ataxia Disruption of bodily movements.

Autoclaving Complete destruction of micro-organisms using steam and pressure. Autoclaving sterilises devices and instruments.

Catheter A probe (tube) made of metal, glass, plastic or rubber, which is inserted into organs of the body (bladder, stomach) for the purposes of emptying, administration of medicines, flushing or examination.

Colostrum The milk produced by the mother in the first few days after birth. Contains high levels of special antibodies, fat-soluble vitamins (vitamins A and D) and trace elements (copper, zinc, iron) and is vitally important for the newborn animal.

Disinfection The use of chemicals to target and destroy undesirable micro-organisms.

Early pregnancy The first half of pregnancy.

Ectoparasites External parasites such as sheep lice, biting lice and mites, which can settle on the outside of a host animal.

Empty Empty dams are non-pregnant dams e.g. between lambing and their next service or found to be no longer pregnant when due to give birth.

Endoparasites Internal parasites such as lungworms, gastrointestinal worms, tapeworms and liver fluke which can settle inside a host animal.

Immune system The body's defence system, including certain organs which produce proteins and defensive cells to protect against infectious diseases.

Infection Entry (active or passive) of pathogenic micro-organisms (viruses, bacteria, fungal organisms, parasites) into a host animal, where they settle and multiply.

Intramuscular (i.m.) Administration of medicines into a muscle.

Intravenous (i.v.) Administration of medicines into a vein.

Lamb feeder Lambs being reared without their mothers are given milk replacer powder, mixed with water, as a cold or warm drink via buckets with rubber teats or semi- or fully automated machines.

Lambing pen Special pen for lambing and the first few days afterwards, fenced off from the rest of the flock.

Late pregnancy The last third of pregnancy.

Lethargy Listlessness, reluctance to move.

Oral Administration of medicines or substances by mouth.

pH Measure of the concentration of hydrogen ions in a solution, used to determine its acidity or alkalinity.

Prepatent period Time between ingestion (infection) of a parasite and the excretion of parasite eggs or larvae in the faeces.

Reflex Involuntary reaction to an external stimulus (e.g. suckling reflex).

Resistance Ability of micro-organisms (bacteria, parasites) to withstand the effects of medicines.

Return to oestrus Female animals come back into heat 16 to 19 days after mating.

Tetracycline An antibiotic drug.

Toxins Poisonous substances produced by plants, animals, bacteria or fungal organisms, or found in the environment.

Vaccine Drug derived from live or killed pathogens which can be used in humans and animals to induce the production of specific antibodies (vaccination).

References

Dedié, K., Bostedt, H. (1996): Schaf- und Ziegenkrankheiten, 2nd ed., Ulmer, Stuttgart.

Dunn, P. (1987): The Goatkeepers Veterinary Book. Farming Press, Ipswich.

Gall, C. F. (2001): Ziegenzucht, 2nd ed., Ulmer, Stuttgart.

Henderson, D. C. (1991): The Veterinary Book for Sheep Farmers. Farming Press, Ipswich.

Korn, S. von (2001): Schafe in Koppel- und Hütehaltung, 2nd ed., Ulmer, Stuttgart.

Loeffler, K. (2002): Anatomie und Physiologie der Haustiere, 10th ed., Ulmer, Stuttgart.

Mayer, A., Scheunemann, H. (1992): Infektionsschutz der Tiere. Hoffmann, Berlin.

Nickel, R., Schummer, A., Seiferle, E. (2003): Lehrbuch der Anatomie der Haustiere, vol. IV, 4th ed., Parey, Berlin, Hamburg.

Späth, H., Thume, O., Wenzler, J.-G. (2012): Ziegen halten, 6th ed., Umer, Stuttgart.

Strittmatter, K. (2004): Schafzucht. Ulmer, Stuttgart.

Stünzi, H., Weiss, E. (1982): Allgemeine Pathologie. Parey, Berlin.

Walser, K., Bostedt, H. (1990): Neugeborenen- und Säuglingskunde der Tiere. Enke, Stuttgart.

Strobel, H. (2009) Klauenpflege Schaf und Ziege, Ulmer, Stuttgart.

Winkelmann, J., Ganter, U. (2008): Farbatlas Schaf- und ZIegenkrankheiten, Ulmer, Stuttgart.

Addresses

Refer to APHA laboratories, and a number of private diagnostic labs in the UK. SRUC labs in Scotland and DARD in Northern Ireland. Farmers are best to contact their own vet if a post mortem is needed or to submit samples.

Index

www.ingramcontent.com/pod-product-compliance
Ingram Content Group UK Ltd.
Pitfield, Milton Keynes, MK11 3LW, UK
UKHW050148280726
14058UKWH00008B/690